NURSE ABUSE
IMPACT AND RESOLUTION

Editors

Laura Gasparis RN, MA, CEN, CCRN
Joan Swirsky RN, MS, CS

with
Ten Contributing Authors

I

Library of Congress catalog card number: 90-91915
ISBN 0-9627246-0-2

Editors: Laura Gasparis RN, MA, CEN, CCRN
Joan Swirsky RN, MS, CS

Design and Production Coordination: Dezigns of Staten Island

Printed in the United States of America

Published by
Power Publications
56 McArthur Avenue
Staten Island, New York 10312
1-800-331-6534

7 6 5 4 3 2 1

Table of Contents

Preface   Laura Gasparis RN, MA, CEN, CCRN
                         Joan Swirsky RN, MS, CS

Chapter 1 pg. 1   **Nursework ... The Reality**
                         Robert G. Hess, Jr. RN, MSN, CCRN, CNA

Chapter 2 pg. 27   **The Present State of Nursing:**
                         Statistics, Economics, Internal Conflicts and
                         Other Obstacles
                         Theresa Mastrorilli RN, BSN, CCRN

Chapter 3 pg. 65   **Forms of Nurse Abuse**
                         Donna Shea Leear RN, BSN, CCRN
                         Cathy Odorisio RN, BSN

Chapter 4 pg. 111   **Historical Perspectives on Nurse Abuse:**
                         How It All Started
                         Susan Giampietro RN, MS, Ph.D (Cand)
                         Joy Schloton-Elwell RN, MS

Chapter 5 pg. 125   **Nurses' Perceptions of Their Hospital Experiences**
                         Judy Carlson-Catalano RN, Ed.D.

Chapter 6 pg. 175   **The Psychology of Abuse**
                         Joan Swirsky RN, MS, CS

Chapter 7 pg. 211   **Another Look At Burnout**
                         Kathy McMahon RN, MSN

Chapter 8 pg. 237   **Nursework: From The Eyes of A Nurse Manager**
                         Camille Silvetti RN, MSN, CCRN

Chapter 9 pg. 253   **Solutions**
                         Joan Swirsky RN, MS, CS

Chapter 10 pg. 293 **Nurse's Bill of Rights**
                         Laura Gasparis RN, MA, CEN, CCRN
                         Donna Shea Leear RN, BSN, CCRN
                         Theresa Mastrorilli RN, BSN, CCRN

About the Authors

Laura Gasparis RN, MA, CEN, CCRN is a critical care consultant who lectures extensively on critical care and medical-surgical nursing. She has held the positions of assistant professor of nursing, staff development instructor and staff nurse and has over eighteen years of experience in critical care nursing. She is presently a per diem staff nurse. Laura is also the owner of Power Publications, a publishing company and president/publisher of A.D. Von Publishers, Inc., publisher of *Revolution - The Journal Of Nurse Empowerment*. She is also the proprietor and director of Education Enterprises, a nursing seminar company. Laura has authored, co-authored and edited a total of ten books such as *Critical Care Examination Review* and *Emergency Nursing Examination Review*, and is the series editor of a six volume *State Board Review Series* published by Springhouse Corporation.

Joan Swirsky RN, MS, CS is a clinical nurse specialist in psychotherapy, as well as an A.S.P.O. certified childbirth educator. Ms. Swirsky, a feature and science writer for the *Womans Record*, a monthly Long Island magazine, is the recipient of five Long Island Press awards. She also writes for *The New York Times, Newsday*, and a variety of magazines. A former editor for Princeton Educational Publishers, she has been editor-in-chief of *The Caucus Current*, a nationally distributed news magazine for the past nine years. Ms. Swirsky's musical, "Oh Baby!", was performed off-off Broadway in 1983. As the book and lyric writer of three additional musicals, she has just completed her first screenplay. Ms. Swirsky is the editor-in-chief of *Revolution - The Journal Of Nurse Empowerment*, a quarterly journal published by A.D. Von Publishers, Inc.

Robert G. Hess, Jr. RN, MSN, CCRN, CNA is currently pursuing full-time doctoral studies in nursing administration at the University of Pennsylvania, while working as a bedside critical care nurse. Bob has an undergraduate in comparative religion from Temple University, a nursing diploma from Frankford Hospital in Philadelphia and a master's in nursing administration from Seton Hall University. He is certified both in critical care and in nursing administration. Bob has extensive management experience in roles from head nurse to director in critical, emergency and skilled nursing care. He has taught graduate nursing administration. Bob is a third degree black belt instructor in karate and kung-fu.

Theresa Mastrorilli RN, BSN, CCRN has been a registered nurse for six years. She is currently employed as a clinical nurse III on staff in a Boston Hospital's critical care unit.

Donna Shea Leear RN, BSN, CCRN has been a staff nurse in the intensive care unit of a community hospital in Boston for eight years. She is also the proprietor of an education seminar company called Shea Associates.

Cathy Odorisio RN, BSN is currently enrolled in an MSN program at Wagner College, Staten Island, New York. She is presently nurse care coordinator in a large university affiliated medical center's neuro-science unit. Cathy has worked actively in nursing for nine years including travel nursing. She has been in a management position for six years.

Susan Giampietro RN, MSN, Ph.D (Cand.) is an instructor of nursing at Lehman College, City University of New York. She has been a medical-surgical clinician within a large medical center.

Joy Schloton-Elwell RN, MSN earned her bachelor's degree in nursing from Long Island University and her Masters degree in nursing from Herbert H. Lehman College, New York. Her areas of practice include critical care as well as medical-surgical nursing. She teaches in several baccalaureate nursing programs in Westchester County, New York, where she lives with her husband and two children.

Judy Carlson-Catalano RN, Ed.D. is on faculty at The College of Staten Island, Staten Island, New York. She is an assistant professor of nursing and is coordinator of research in nursing and issues in nursing courses. Judy also teaches leadership in nursing practice, physical assessment, health throughout the life cycle and medical-surgical nursing. Current research interests include power in nursing practice and coping with chronic illness. She has presented internationally, nationally and locally on power and empowerment.

Kathleen McMahon RN, MSN is a registered nurse with a Master of science from Adelphi University. Kathy is currently a clinical instructor with The College of Staten Island, Staten Island, New York and a practicing critical care nurse.

Camille Silvetti RN, MSN, CCRN was an assistant director of nursing for critical care at Flushing Hospital Medical Center in New York. Presently a nursing coordinator in a large medical center, Camille has ten years of experience in nursing administration.

Preface

In every society throughout history, nursing has been practiced. In birth, in growth, in health and in illness — as human beings mature, grow old and ultimately prepare to die, certain individuals are universally sought out to care for, to *nurse* others.

Today, health-related moral and ethical concerns have become more complex. The AIDS crisis presents the healthcare community with challenges and dangers perhaps unprecedented in history. Diagnostic techniques have become increasingly sophisticated and treatment regimes more technologically advanced. As the human life span continues to be prolonged at both ends of the continuum, the need, indeed the *demand* for superior and more humane healthcare has increased as never before.

Nowhere is this need more keenly felt than in the realm of *nursing care.* As we stand at the threshold of a new century, the need for highly skilled, technically proficient and professionally educated nurses is greater than at any other time in history. This is particularly felt in the acute care hospital setting where patients are released from hospitals sooner therefore increasing the need for quality nursing care in the home setting as well.

Why has this need progressively arisen? With almost 2 million registered nurses in the United States, why is there an escalating demand for more of them? Why is the healthcare system faced with a situation in which the very care of the hospitalized patient is increasingly compromised? In essence: *Why the nursing shortage?*

The present nursing shortage has a multitude of causes including: deficiencies in the healthcare reimbursement system; diminished nursing school enrollment as women seek more lucrative professional opportunities elsewhere, and, on the heels of the latest technological advancements is the increased demand for professional nurses.

The focus of this book concerns itself with an additional factor — one that is often alluded to, but rarely confronted head-on — **NURSE ABUSE.**

The diminishing number of staff nurses at the bedside compromises the attention and care that every patient has the right to expect. Nurses are recruited from foreign countries in which culture, education and language differences may ill-equip them to occupy positions within the healthcare settings of this country. And, as a harbinger of even greater problems affecting the healthcare of future generations, nursing school enrollment has declined precipitously.

There is some irony here — for never before has the population of registered nurses been better equipped, academically and clinically, to tend to the population's healthcare needs. Nurses are very versatile professionals. With preparation in the sciences of psychology and pathology, proficiency in assessment skills and knowledge of preventative care, they possess the ability to apply this knowledge to clinical practice. This body of knowledge, combined with a background in the social and behavioral sciences, sets nurses apart from other health disciplines. This unique combination of knowledge and expertise enables nurses to assume broad responsibilities in all aspects of healthcare including teaching, liaison work, community outreach, and administration. These are the characteristics of the modern nurse.

The versatility of the professional nurse has made his or her contribution essential in managing the day-to-day operation of major healthcare institutions in this country. In fact, nurses comprise the only professional presence "around the clock" in both hospitals and nursing homes. They play a vital role, as their astuteness in clinical assessment, their anticipation of impending crisis, and their care-taking capacities are essential to the well being of their patients. Furthermore, nurses have direct accountability for the nursing care that they deliver day after day.

And yet, in spite of their excellent preparation and society's need for their services, they are abandoning hospital life in great numbers, leaving the explanation for this phenomenon to the theories of social scientists, hospital administrators and distressed nursing academics. Even while local and national classified pages carry columns of want ads offering nurses employment, nurses are leaving the profession of nursing.

How do these theoreticians explain what has become the preeminent issue in the healthcare system? Depending on their perspective, their explanations run the gamut. Although data indicates that nurses who experience "job satisfaction" do not place salary as the first or most important criterion, the most common theory used to explain the nursing shortage is that nurses are finally fed up with receiving wages that challenge the lowest end of the pay scale. While it is true that many nurses have sought career opportunities which yield greater economic rewards, the reason for their defection, unfortunately, cannot be solely attributed to economic motives.

Others cite the increased opportunity for nurses to practice independently as midwives, psychotherapists, teachers, pediatric specialists, etc. And still others express the notion that the aspirations of a new "feminist" mentality have inspired women (it is important to remember here that 97% of nurses are women) to seek avenues of employment which are more empowering. Other factors which attempt to explain this critical problem include the devalued position of women in society, the disproportionate authority and dominance of physicians and the stressful hospital environment.

Again, while it is true that many nurses feel powerless to effect change within their work setting, and while it is also true that they resent some of the inflexible working conditions, these age-old issues and circumstances alone cannot account for the current crisis. While these factors may be symptomatic of the problems which have evolved in nursing, virtually from its inception, the underlying cause of this widespread exodus is **NURSE ABUSE.**

The pervasive abuse of nurses permeates a system which begins with their academic preparation and clinical training, and continues in the settings, all settings, in which nurses work.

Undervalued, subject to the most ancient and pernicious stereotypes, and treated with cavalier indifference or crass condescension, nurses are now beginning to echo the sentiments of the movie hero who, in despair and disgust, exclaimed, "I'm fed up and I'm not going to take it anymore!" Everyone has their figurative "bottom line", the point beyond which they cannot be pushed. In the nursing community, the bottom line has been unusually flexible, ever accommodating to the indignities, insults and shabby treatment which few others would abide. The nursing shortage, which has now gripped the country with health emergencies and desperate contingency plans, is a clear indication that nurses, too, will "not take it anymore."

Unfortunately, across the country, nurses are expressing their grievances quite dramatically — they leave nursing. But wherever and whenever we raised the issue of **NURSE ABUSE** or expressed the intention of publishing a book on this subject, nurses have responded enthusiastically

— happy that, at last, their story will be told. "I'll write it!" some have said. "Send me a dozen copies," others exclaim. "When can I get my hands on a copy?" "I want to send one to my professor, supervisor, director, attending doctor ..." No one asked for the expression **NURSE ABUSE** to be explained or defined — the note of recognition that it elicited was truly remarkable, as if embodied within those two words was a universal truth which made further definition unnecessary.

"NURSE ABUSE: IMPACT AND RESOLUTION" is a compilation of essays that are the authors' personal reflection of a profession in crisis. It represents a combined effort of staff nurses, nurse administrators, professors of nursing and nurse researchers who focused on some of the special issues, problems and barriers confronting nurses, as well as offering possible solutions. Our intention in publishing this book is twofold: To provide a forum through which the perceptions, concerns and frustrations of the abused professional nurse can be presented and to provide possible solutions for our profession.

Bringing the subject of **NURSE ABUSE** out of the proverbial closet where it has been isolated and unaddressed for too long, is the first step toward a critical self-analysis by nurses. This must take place if the noble art and science of nursing is to claim its rightful and respected place in the healthcare system. As editors, it is our fervent hope that this book will act as a catalyst for a long overdue and meaningful change.

Laura Gasparis RN, MA, CEN, CCRN
Joan Swirsky RN, MS, CS

Acknowledgments

The development and writing of this book was truly a collective venture by a wonderful group of dedicated nurses. This book owes its existence to many people.

It was at dinner with Donna Shea Leear and Theresa Mastrorilli that the idea of Nurse Abuse: Impact and Resolution was conceived. Thank you for lighting the spark.

Sincere appreciation is extended to all the contributing authors for expressing themselves both personally and professionally. Their work is insightful, inspiring, and at times painful but all necessary for the critical analysis and awareness needed in our profession.

Throughout the writing of this book, many nurses became interested and provided their ideas, feedback, support and encouragement. Our gratitude to Ginny Kottkamp RN, MS, CNM for her painstaking statistical analysis and to Marion Kinsella LPN, who kept the ink flowing in Cathy's pen.

We like to extend a loving gratitude to Fay Gasparis, whose constant nurturing, support and secretarial expertise have made this possible. Sincere and special appreciation to our two best friends — our husbands, Charles and Steven. Thank you for standing by our side.

We are indebted to David Foil from DLP and Carol Weiss for their work as copy editors. Their advice, interest and editing were extremely helpful.

We were also fortunate to have a great deal of support from some extraordinary people. Ann and Dave Navarria are special friends who played an integral part in the production of this book. Together, with the help of staff member Roseann Foley, this book became a reality. They were enthusiastic and ever so creative.

Our deepest appreciation to all.

L.G.
J.S.

Chapter One

Nursework... The Reality

I can't imagine the American hospital system without nurses — and neither can the American public. Daily hospital confusion goes something like this: Patient to any passing woman: "Nurse, I need you." Passing woman: "I'm not the nurse; I'm the housekeeper." Patient to next passing women: "Nurse. Nurse! I need to talk to you." Next passing women: "I'm not your nurse; I'm the dietary worker ... the social worker ... the respiratory therapist ... the nurses aide ... the pharmacy aide." Crowds of healthcare workers seem to get larger, nurses seem to get fewer, and these chosen few are simply being abused.

American hospital patients are nurse-junkies; just put Americans in a hospital and immediately they want "their" nurses. But nurses are a shared phenomenon, a vital resource necessary for the nation's health, but carelessly squandered by a desperate and aging America. Our nation is so accustomed to unlimited gratification of its needs that an inadequate supply of nurses seems incomprehensible to most Americans. Nurses are hard to find these days, especially in hospitals. Nurses are leaving hospital practice every day. Underpaid, overworked, not respected, and finally insulted, they leave to practice elsewhere. Some take transient home healthcare jobs, often the last stop in nursing for burnt-out hospital nurses. Buried by paper work, which must be completed to document and justify the adequacy and appropriateness of their patient care, they bail out altogether.

There are almost two million nurses practicing the art and science — the *mystery* — of nursing, in the United States. Further mystery lies in their motivation, their energy for caring, and their unbounded expertise in science and technology. There are all the trappings of a separate culture in this group, or perhaps of a major religion — the "cult of caring." In every form of healthcare, physical or mental, you can find these people scurrying around, risking sanity, exceeding their physical capacity, and risking their self-esteem on a daily basis. There is great news about this group — and also some bad. The public has been subjected to a negative "press" regarding the nursing situation and this mandates close examination by a nurse. First, here's some reality.

The dwindling fuel for the profession these days comes from young people who have considered all risks and options, adolescents who have never wanted to do anything else, women and men in their second careers and humanists still capable of caring for humanity, all responding to the same idealistic lure. At great personal cost, they continue in their mission of nursing care, freely providing that care to whomever asks for it. At the hub of human existence, nurses become the fail-safe mechanism of healthcare; when they fail, the health system fails.

Another National Nurses Day just passed in May, and the happy celebrations of hospital nursing departments concealed a grim reality. Typically represented by thousands of dollars of classified newspaper ads, Nurses Day futilely summoned nurses to hospital employment with graphic flash and hype. Nurses Day obscured a "Great American Nurse Buy-Out." Incentives in the form of cars,

Caribbean cruises, tuition pay-offs (a new form of inden-
tured servitude), and even bounties for ransoming fellow
nursing colleagues to healthcare agencies exploded in full-
page ads. Euphemistically listed under "Medical Opportunities," the real game afoot was to entice unsuspecting
nurses to certain doom — hospital employment. The bigger the advertisement, the greater the risk.

All this clutter expressed the classier side of recruitment. Hot competition for new graduate nurses has led
nurse recruiters into their own reality, a kind of tribal
consciousness. As a discrete group, these nurses convene
in "recruitment fairs" to shower new nurses with chants
and incantations, venerating their respective hospitals as
new planes of cosmic employment. Blatant misrepresentation is so often the rule that one must assume that these
"nurse dealers" must all have learned their trade on the
same used-car lot. When the rattles and incense fail, the
recruiters attempt to buy the new graduates with coffee
mugs and pens. This is their not so subtle message: We
offer trinkets to the village idiots.

In the excitement and pursuit, some hospitals have
stopped reference checks. The sole credential for eligibil-
ity, it seems, has become simply having two legs! This
grim state of affairs is not universal, but is concentrated
in the "combat pay" hospitals of American cities. My hospital has stopped most formal newspaper advertising since
it has become embarrassing to broadcast such severity of
need (and it hasn't worked anyway).

Nursing executives have succumbed to a rather du-
bious solution to the nursing shortage. For immediate relief, they now entice nurses from any country, plundering
other nations of their own nursing resources. It is told to
the nursing staff that it's more economical to import than
to advertise, and thus the staff perceives that one would
rather look for cheaper alternatives than to invest money

in our underpaid American nurses. Nurses with green cards, trapped in modern, short-term quasi-bondage, camouflage the critical shortage by inserting their foreign bodies into vacant nursing positions. By paying an experienced foreign nurse the same entry level wages as a new American nurse, some administrators perpetuate the same low nursing wages that discourage more Americans from entering the profession. **NURSE ABUSE.**

Foreign nurses can be excellent practitioners in their own lands, but their educational systems are often different from those of American-trained nurses. American nurses are trained as generalists, while foreign nurses are often restricted within a specialty early in training; these nurses do not share our common nursing language or proficiency in the English language. But mere mastery of the spoken word pales beside the necessary mastery of the complex cultural nuances and diverse mores of heterogeneous America. Bicultural nursing, or meeting the needs of various cultures within the United States itself, has presented challenge enough to American nurses without staffing our hospitals with other country's cultures. Are we selling out our own? As we invade Ireland, England, and the Philippines for more nurses, are we selling out our own?

Emergency room nurses are taught that although disasters come in all sizes, they have one common thread: inadequate resources to meet an emergent need. In disasters, "you do the best you can."

Unlimited access to healthcare no longer being considered a privilege reserved for the affluent alone, Americans have identified a national need for nursing in astonishing proportions. They have decided that perpetual health is the right of every human being who resides in America; but they are not willing to pay for it. Americans, with their sense of entitlement, have increasingly demanded that American nurses subsidize this typically American choice for anything bigger and better with lower salaries and higher productivity than the rest of the nation's workers. As American nurses feel this increasing demand at their backs, they are responding with their feet: by walking away. Nurses' compensation is simply not equitable. And recognition of their valued contribution is woefully inadequate ... so, nurses are leaving the profession. Years of acquired skill and experience are flushed away without a single sigh from the motherland.

There are no catastrophic waves when a single nurse leaves her practice. No newspaper advertisement announces her departure; no national wailing ensues, and no one has suggested the creation of Nurse Memorial Day. But there are cumulative effects insinuating themselves into everyday healthcare reality. Hospitals increasingly resort to "diversion," a dangerous new practice for the '90s. Diversion occurs when emergency rooms are closed to selected admissions as a result of an absence of available hospital beds because there are no nurses to staff them. Diversion is like a pinball game in an arcade where the ball careens from bumper to bumper, sometimes collecting points, but ultimately seeking the reward of an exit from the game. However, the pinball in this case is an ambulance carrying a human life in mortal danger; the streets are not a game, but a means to an end. The bumpers are the closed emergency entrances to hospitals housing expensive technology and all the refinements of modern medical science. The benefits of miraculous medicine are worthless to this human encased in a traveling wheeled pinball if EDs are closed to him; any "right" to emergent care becomes simply meaningless if unavailable. Without nurses, there is no portal to healthcare — no emergency room, no critical care unit, no hospital. The doctors can doctor all they want, but without nurses, the system cannot serve its clientele in any way.

Society simply keeps asking for more from our colleagues who are becoming fewer and fewer. We are hoping against hope that there will be a nurse around for our own parents and our own family members as time goes on. As nurses, we keep "rearranging our priorities" and "meeting the patients' real, not self-perceived needs." This is all jargon in "nursespeak" for rationalizing why we can't provide the nursing care we were once educated to provide — the care we could take such pride in rendering. There just aren't enough of us to provide all the care that is both expected and demanded, and so the bureaucrats of America would have us lower our standards. Nurses won't do that. They'd rather leave their profession.

Nurses work tirelessly around the clock, around the calendar: all shifts, including holidays and weekends. And they work wherever they are sent. In hospitals, we complement each other's work (functional nursing), get together and knock off the work like a flying squadron (team nursing), sweat it out in solitude with our little group of patients (primary nursing) or choreograph care-like little business enterprises (case management nursing). We've used ingenious tricks to get the job done; but we've been so clever that the nation thinks we can keep this up forever. I don't think we can.

Nurses' current bid for survival is to delegate their bedside nursing tasks, and therefore some of the art that *is* bedside nursing, to others. This is not easily done, but probably necessary. We know that few would sanction paying over $30,000 per year to someone who routinely provides bed baths — and yet, it's what the professional nurse brings to the bed bath — in terms of specialized assessment skills and advanced scientific knowledge — that makes such an expenditure a good investment. Nurses are criticized both for staying away from the bedside and for spending too much time at the bedside. A physician recently complained that nurses had deteriorated over the last few years. He challenged, "I've told other nursing directors before you and now I'm telling you. When I come on the unit these days, I can never find a nurse. I'll bet they're in with the patients, bathing them, writing about them, holding their hands. God knows what they're doing, but I know what they should be doing. They should be at the desk so I can make rounds. I know, because I'm married to a nurse." ["Rounds" is often the act of transcribing nurses' meticulously gathered data into their own progress notes as if they had obtained it first hand.] I was speechless, but thought, "How arrogant! The nurse to whom he's married hasn't nursed for twenty years; she doesn't know what the nurses do. The nurses are with their patients and this guy is upset about it."

As professionals, nurses frequently rely on the examples of their mentors, eliciting their past learning and remembering the experienced advice of their mentors to guide them in the practice of their craft. My most unforgettable nursing instructor was from an earlier era in nursing who practiced the profession as an art form. Her most amazing, yet consistent, accomplishment was to make sick people feel better. Sometimes she just turned them from side to side in bed, other times she just smiled, touching them or talking compassionately; her patients always felt better when she left them. As a student, this was rather mysterious and maddening to me. As I devoured the nursing knowledge base as quickly as I could and soon absorbed its science, this art form eluded me for many years. When I practice bedside nursing now, I try to summon the instructor's magic to help my patients feel better and cared for. I watch nurses with this magic struggle for its effect everyday, always without the necessary time to feel its effect.

To the uninitiated, basic nursing care seems to be a series of little jobs of varying complexity. Basic nursing seems to be tasks, like taking temperature and blood pressure readings or administering medications. But these visible parts belie the sophisticated whole. Every physical act in nursing is the manifestation of a cognitive process which incorporates assessment, planning, implementation, and evaluation of nursing care. A nurse's thought process involves continuous observation of a patient's response to his body and mind, the internal environment, and his surroundings, the external environment. This is the basic arena for what nurses call the nursing process, a sophisticated problem-solving approach for the scientific analysis of the complicated open system, man and his environment. Through this process a nurse synthesizes subsequent nursing actions, basic or otherwise.

Basic nursing is composed of mandatory nursing actions relating to a patient's most basic needs. For example, if no other care is given, nurses must meet the survival needs of their patients by providing the essential care for hygiene, nutrition, elimination, sleep and so on. Unfortunately, the current healthcare situation dictates that nurses accomplish basics at the expense of subtle ritual ingredients, like a nurse's presence with a patient in pain, that would make the human difference in patient outcomes. The nurses know that they should do more for their patients, but cannot. Although empirically grounded in both the "hard" and "soft" sciences, nurses would also practice a very human science to guide their patients to a successful outcome. When nurses are short-staffed, their practice is often reduced to the "basics" and the potential of this wonderful blend of science and art form is not realized. Nurses' high self-expectations do not accept any justification for not realizing this potential, making their own frustration with this overwhelming.

I wonder what nursing would be like if there were no nurses who remembered the art form. Today there are several categories of ancillary nursing personnel, like nurse aides, nursing assistants, orderlies and technicians who, by performing tedious basic nursing tasks, extend the care (and responsibility) of the professional nurse to a greater number of patients. As nurses are forced to delegate basic tasks and precious opportunities for face-to-face caring are left to non-professional care-givers or nurse-extenders, what will become of the "essence" of the profession? Who will do the caring? Who will make the patients feel better? Nurses' biggest charge will be to teach the science to their extenders. But how will we teach the art form? And how can we possibly teach experience?

Hospitals are now trying to hire greater numbers of nurses aides to compensate for RN staffing shortages. The state boards of nursing are in dispute over what these people can and will be able to do. A few years ago no one really cared about delineating the aides' activities when there was an adequate supply of nurses or, as many wrongfully assumed, too many RNs. Then, aides could perform just about any task that the nurses felt they could handle, given sufficient teaching and supervision. Now some out-of-touch regulatory boards are worried about resultant quality of care if non-professional caregivers happen to perform "complex" nursing tasks — like enemas. One state regulatory agency played host to the "Great Enema Controversy." Countless debates raged throughout the state between a bureaucratic agency and nursing service administrators, all questioning the wisdom of home health aides performing a thankless task which has been delivered by anyone's mother for years. The board's final edict: only licensed personnel should stick tubes in people's rectums. The consumer is once again protected.

I suggest that such regulatory agents should annually work mandated time as staff in the agencies they purport to evaluate; let them listen to the staff as they work. A little reality would certainly shore up their shaky credibility.

Quality of care has been traditionally controlled by the nurses in practice (as they practice) and not by regulatory bodies. Perhaps someone has confused the nurses aides with the disease. What nurses aides really are is the cheapest labor force in American hospitals, but not the most cost-effective. Like most nursing personnel, they can only legally function in the presence of a registered professional nurse; the safety of their performance is a measure of a supervising nurse's liability. Even though they are now called nursing assistants, a weekly news magazine recently listed their job as one of the ten worst jobs in the nation; the survey did not discuss the methodology for this pronouncement. Nursing assistants are currently trained on the job and must be supervised. Nurses carefully devise work assignments for the aides, monitor their progress and evaluate the results. It can be wearisome business for both parties, and the professional nurse finds herself responsible and liable for the outcomes of the aides' work. A nurse can feel comfortable delegating "non-nursing" tasks, like filling water pitchers, running to other departments as a courier, transporting patients, posting lab reports or delivering food trays. However, her margin of comfort tends to decrease when assigning essential bedside nursing practice to a minimally trained aide. Mistakes in monitoring a patient's vital signs, especially when life-supporting drug infusions are altered based on the data, can be devastating to the patient's progress in life. Nurses generally hold themselves to a standard of 100% accuracy and expect it from each other. The error of a subordinate could easily trigger a nurse's flight from the profession. Nurses care that much.

One hundred percent accuracy is not a common human standard. Nurses have fooled themselves into thinking that they can achieve this with unfailing repetition. When a physician commits an error, it is termed a "complication." A nurse generally offers her head on a platter to the general public for any error, however minor. Hospitals used to paternalistically protect nurses like any other hospital employee under the umbrella of the institution's insurance carrier. Now, a hospital's insurance carrier will defend a nurse against a patient-initiated suit and then sue their own nurse for any error of judgment to recoup any financial losses from the initial litigation. Nurses' malpractice insurance costs do not match those of the physicians, but the annual percentage increases, specialty by specialty, are becoming comparable.

I still wonder why, in the face of an extreme nursing shortage, the public doesn't question a situation where half of a nurse's duties are still "non-nursing" tasks. When I was a relatively well-paid nursing supervisor in an urban teaching hospital, we used to joke about my status as an expensive courier. One of my duties was to take pre-operative patients' false teeth to a safe in the nursing office so they didn't get lost. A nurse's precious time is sometimes abused to solve the most stupid problems.

In the midst of all this controversy, the better nurses tell me that if they could pick a profession all over again, they'd still become nurses and even encourage their children to get involved. One of the finest aspects about being a nurse is that you get to spend your time with other nurses, exceptionally fine folk. You get to witness fellow human beings acting with compassion and altruism on behalf of strangers on a daily basis. You routinely participate in heroics that are the stuff of great novels, grand dreams and lofty religions. Nurses never talk about religion, they practice it. When I asked a staff nurse if her religion influenced her practice, she told me that she treated every patient as though he was Christ. That's pretty heady stuff and she meant it. Can you imagine how wonderful it would be if all people lived by such values in 20th century America?

Nurses are involved in the sincere care of every conceivable aspect of life and death. Yet nurses are so busy doing nursing that they don't take the time to talk about it. We have allowed other people to define our practice for years and that is perhaps the greatest abuse of nurses. Instead of using the media, we have allowed our abuse by them. Media routinely depict nurses as mother, nymph or whore, depending on the morality of the era; this is pap for the public and, unfortunately, nurses have never taken this seriously. But the output of assertive nurse authors is attacking this situation.

Hospitals turn a profit and the administrators take the credit; but hospitals often remain solvent because of criminally cheap nursing salaries. A patient gets better and the physicians claim the success; but nurses have known for years that many diseases progress along a course all of their own, regardless of medical intervention. Often, patients get better because of the medical care suggested to inexperienced resident physicians by the nurses. Sometimes the best that can be offered to a patient is the support of nursing care; thus, successful medical outcomes are sometimes the result of nursing care. Nursing has been misrepresented on so many fronts that we're in danger of this faulty image becoming the new reality. We are close to becoming the victim the media have portrayed.

Nurses have consistently made such differences in the lives of Americans and this must be articulated in as many ways. When I told my friends that I had hired nursing assistants to give patients their physical care —

the beds and baths, the bedpans and urinals, the tasks no one would ever think of doing in a white uniform — my friends wondered just what the nurses would do with additional time on their hands. And so, it became obvious to me that even my friends had mistakenly equated a collection of simple tasks with a national resource — our nurses. Likewise, the American public routinely missed the invisible, but vital "soft" stuff that nurses provide but never market. Nurses have quietly slipped into the background of everyone's life, catching babies and burying relatives, figuratively and literally. Nurses are simply a celebration of life, a confrontation with death, and a support for everything in between.

I am not angry with America for displacing the recognition and compensation nurses deserve to other professions. We as nurses haven't bothered to explain our practice to each other, let alone the public. We have just kept working, working shorter and cheaper, working longer. We're in crisis now and this crisis demands our own introspection, and articulation, and action. America needs to know why we're worth preserving, why we're so needed and why we might cost more these days.

Everyone has had a nurse in his or her life who was sorely needed at the time; everyone needs a nurse sometime. America, your nurse is an impression softly but permanently etched in your mind over the last twenty years. America, your nurse was there, absolutely, without judgment and without reservation, when you were in need. Nurses are all over the place in roles that you expect and also in many unexpected ones.

Just to jar your memory a bit, I'd like to remind you of your nurse:
• Remember when you delivered your first-born and you felt too shy to hold him? That delivery was the result of meticulous vigilance and intervention by some of nursing's

finest scientists, the delivery room nurses. They monitored the progress of you and your child and applied their skills to nature's course whenever necessary to insure a favorable outcome. Subsequent children were born and you looked for a standard to guide you appropriately as a mother. It was a nurse who found time to teach you to touch the child, to accept your awkward feelings and to relay what is not really inherited: the nurse would teach you to parent. Nurses in the delivery room, the nursery and the post-partum unit would offer their expertise, acquired through the synthesis of anatomy, physiology, psychology and other sciences, all related to the birthing process. A nurse would take a step beyond her academic foundation. She would even become a role model, if that's what you needed.

• Later, one after the other, your children would begin to walk, taking the steps that would eventually lead them away to their own worlds and their own children. But every time they fell or faltered, you would worry, "Is this all right? Are they normal?" Your concern went beyond legs, steps and balance, and you wanted assurance that the whole child was well. You asked the nurse, holistically grounded in theories of normal growth and development and family systems, the only professional who was qualified to recognize what is normal. She would examine your child, his friends, his family; she would consider both the person and the environment. She might tell you not to fix what is not broken.

• While your children grew, you might have had a friend or a neighbor, someone who was a nurse. She always seemed available for a chat about the kids and for you. This was not small talk. This was always a serious matter since this nursing person had the professional knowledge to validate your parental observations; she could always tell you how the children were "doing," how they were adjusting to life. You never wondered if such a backyard consultation might be an imposition or why the nurse would continue to speak of nursing concerns. To members of this caring profession, nursing is not a role that ceases beyond the work environment. A nurse is always a nurse, no matter where she is. We, nurses and public, have accepted this.

• Along his way, the child might have become so sick that his care was beyond your capabilities. Your concern, your worry and your love would not be enough; the child needed constant professional nursing care. Incredibly, you were given no alternative but to relinquish custody and control, allowing your child's admission to the company of strangers in a hospital. Though you were fearful, one magic event improved the situation: you met and immediately trusted the nurses and then, you could trust the hospital. Your family's trauma would be alleviated by the nurses.

Although it appeared to be play, the nurses would find something to interest your child, diverting his attention so you could retire home for a spell. The child would be comforted through play and assessed in many ways all the while; evaluating a child's response to health or disease is a part of nursing assessment. Because the focus of nursing encompasses the total person, nurses would take special interest in you as well as the child, never judging, always supporting your own patterns of coping and offering alternate strategies.

• Your life and the lives of those you love progress constantly, merging on a continuum of relationships which constitute your daily reality until the abrupt shock of a major calamity occurs. Crises visit a family in many and usually unexpected ways: a car or household accident, a minor sickness turned catastrophic, a chronic condition whirling out of control, or a blast of pain crashing through your chest. As your loved one decompensates in your presence, the advice comes instantly — get him to an Emergency Department. Ambulances wail, heightening urgency and anxiety as you pray for refuge in that haven of care. Swirling amidst chaos, the nurse magically appears again. She might be in her sixteenth hour of work, bludgeoned by a dozen previous cases. She probably had already provided care and comfort for those with several simple injuries, major and minor ailments. But there she is, ready for you and you alone.

The Emergency Department is the antithesis of a controlled environment. It is a window on the world's problems. Sunday mornings are usually the quietest — until "the bus pulls in." Again, as demand outweighs available resources, it is here that a disaster is apt to occur. As several ambulances pull into an already challenged port, the triage nurse will remain attentive to all this stimuli and then focus on the necessary. Your case is pulled to the forefront and the nurse will mobilize the entire healthcare team for your benefit. A physician will be summoned, blood tests obtained, x-rays taken and, if necessary, an appropriate hospital bed secured. You will probably never know that the nurse was just abused by the craziness of a drug addict, that she just sent a child to the morgue, that she has just resuscitated a young heart attack victim's body without being able to save his brain. Her focus at this moment will be on your needs. The tragedies of her shift are processed later, off the job and in her private moments. After this experienced professional washes the blood and guts from a stretcher, changes the linen and readies the room for the next calamity, her years of nursing will pull her through to the next time. But please don't ever mistake a nurse's poise for not caring. Nurses are not hardened to the experience of crisis. They simply learned to translate their caring into action — and you need that now.

• Most people get sick and most, no matter how sick, could be cared for at home if there was adequate available nursing staff. Except for ten minutes of a physician's visit, a day in the hospital stay is about twenty-four hours of nursing care. From the perspective of a hospital nurse, it appears that a hospital stay is an inevitable part of everyone's life. As you spin into this weird and artificial structure, you are inevitably ushered through department after department of little groups of people, all integrated toward two grand goals — the perpetuation of your welfare and that of the institution. How lucky it is for you that when these goals conflict, a nurse will view you as the priority and will be your advocate.

There will be nurses everywhere: medical for acute and chronic conditions, surgical for cutting interventions, critical care for life-threatening events, and specializations reflecting the continuum of life from birth to death. The cult of caring unfolds into subcultures of specialties, all sharing a common body of unique humanistic knowledge, grounded in the latest and most comprehensive advances of science. You might be shuttled through several nursing units, but they are all hubs of coordination for nursing care and support services. The separate units become daily battlegrounds for stress and strain. The nurses will seek responsiveness from themselves and others in this system in order to get you fed, turned and bathed, medicated, medically treated and comforted. They will insure that the pharmacist gets the right orders, that the housekeepers clean your room, and that your telephone and television are turned on.

Your every move and the functioning of the support services will be documented to insure the integrity of your progress and as a record for future use. They might spend up to 40% of their time recording their observations; their commentary is so important that it often becomes the guiding light for your medical care. If she's not in the patient's room, the nurse will be at the desk, writing. Away from the patient, she's easy prey for the troubled family member who asks "How's my mother doing today?" A nurse will stop whatever she's doing, however important, to comfort this family member. She'll also interrupt this ritual documentation for the physician, the housekeeper, her supervisor and especially her patient. When her shift ends, she'll still find herself "charting," knowing that the accuracy of her report is imperative for her patient and for a litigious public.

Always moving, the nurse is omnipresent and under scrutiny. A hospital nurse is always "on" and instantly available to anyone who works or stays in the hospital. There is no private time and often no breaks or meals. A nurse will not allow herself to have a bad day in public, but musters incredible and consistent discipline to care for someone else. She's always only a call bell away from her patients.

Nurses' productivity may be one of the most amazing phenomena in working America. Nurses adjust their work pace to an erratic workload on a 24 hour basis. When the number of patients increase (patient volume) or the patients get sicker (patient acuity), nurses just move and think more quickly. Dealing in human beings, the most variable of creatures, nurses must provide unpredictable amounts of patient care regardless of the available staff. There are no resources waiting in the wings, no instant nurses to strengthen the team. Nurses just work harder.

Some items might be prioritized or relegated to a lesser degree of significance. Maybe breakfast is a half-hour late, medications delayed (with forty patients needing meds at 10 A.M., simultaneous delivery is impossible), or a bath detained. Nurses are very ritualistic and extremely sensitive to a disrupted routine. But the important work gets done. The elderly and dependent receive nourishment and hygiene; only nurses know who on a nursing unit are entirely dependent on nurses for their daily survival and it is those people who receive first attention.

Usually, it is the patients who are well enough to walk and talk who are most apt to notice when the timing of daily nursing care is altered. The American public, raised during a past surplus of nurses who practiced a less sophisticated science, still hold unrealistic expectations of their nurses. Nurses pragmatically shift resources, cutting out those niceties of care which simulate a hotel environment, items inappropriately identified with essential professional nursing care.

No nurse would argue against fresh water, clean linen and a quiet, convalescent surrounding for a patient; these concerns are nursing's heritage from Florence Nightingale. However, even Florence would quickly trash the hotel stuff in the face of a patient's cardiac arrest or the patient who takes a turn for the worse in a less dramatic way. Trust a nurse, she knows where to shift the care. A famous nurse theorist, Dorothea Orem, advocates that a nurse's goal is to restore the client to his highest possible level of independent functioning. Maybe patients who are well enough to walk should get their own water and make their own beds anyway. Nurses know that such activity is often better for their patients. Given the history of American hospital care, nurses are having a difficult time marketing this concept.

As if going to a hospital wasn't enough, just imagine the anxiety associated with the words "critical care." Technology is at its finest here with millions of dollars routinely poured into computerized, physiologic patient monitoring devices. For the average consumer, this sophistication is transformed into incessant beeps, flashes, wails and whining. As the patient turns in bed, another alarm explodes. He thinks, "Is it me? Has my heart gone bad? Did my nurse hear that? Will someone rush in and save me?" Instead, a few minutes later, a nurse wanders into the room to adjust another oversensitive machine and delivers another of countless reassurances: "It's only the monitor, the pump, the respirator; you're okay and we are watching." That's what the critical care nurses are paid for: to wait and watch, positioned for immediate intervention when a critical event tries to snatch your life away. Of course this drama only punctuates the important tasks of maintaining your bodily functions. You still need hygiene and nourishment, but now (in critical care) the nurses may tend devices which breathe for you, evaluating a respirator's function from the gases in your blood. They might calibrate machines that measure pressures and amounts of blood pumped from your heart, titrate drugs which alter the heart's function and monitor machines that even take over your heart's job of pumping. They may track the pressures in your head and even your brain waves. Scary notions, but you're in the best of care. With so much to go wrong and so much to know, critical care units are permeated with the uncertainty of emergency rooms. The patients are there, but the outcomes are unpredictable.

Critical care nurses suffer a constant race with the advances of science. What they know can become hopelessly outdated within a year. Their routine includes a series of catastrophic events, often practicing independent cross-over medicine (yes, they are the doctors' substitutes when physicians are running their offices or sleeping at night). Yet nurses always focus on the whole individual behind the machines. Somehow they can always reach through the tubes and wires to find you. They protect you from getting lost in a jungle of technology amongst a rioting mob of consultants.

When they're done with your care, they switch their skills to your family. Explaining every machine and alarm, they support your family's coping behaviors, whatever they are. If it's your husband who has been trapped into a patient role, and he needs you, they might set up a bed for you to stay by him. They might babysit your children, leave you alone, or even send you home to rest. They'll make telephone calls for you, arrange lodging and deliver messages. They'll appear to stop whatever they're doing to respond to your needs. Poised and ready, they're constantly processing the patient, evaluating physiologic responses to nursing and medical care. In the middle of the night, it's the nurses who stay at the hard-wired bedside with the patient. They decide when the physician should be called, often recommending appropriate therapy before it's medically suggested. If your heart ever stops in a critical care unit, the nurses won't wait for medical advice. It's then or never and you can bet that she'll literally shock (defibrillate) you back to life.

• Nurses are the complete care-givers, focusing on both mind and body. But when the mind, in particular, becomes ill, there is a select group of experts, psychiatric nurses, whose knowledge base is utilized to diagnose and treat emotional trauma or mental disorders.

Living in our modern and complex society, it is not uncommon to be afflicted with depression, fear, anxiety and ineffective coping devices. Mixing rationalizations and delusions in a tired world, people begin to forget what realities they have merely invented and what is really there. Maybe emotional problems or mental illness have visited your spouse, your child or your parents, imposing chaos on the delicate, carefully built relationships that form the substance of your domestic or professional life. Panic leads to further disarray.

The psychiatric nurses can help. Once again, they'll become safe people you can trust as you sort out your thoughts through the therapeutic relationship. Every interaction will be pointed toward a goal of rescue and recovery. They might gradually involve your loved ones in your recovery until your former life is restored, stronger and more insightful. Your friends, your pastor, and any personal support systems will be enlisted for your aid. The final phase will generate strategies to prevent another fall. You're never alone with a nurse.

• Nurses are often lifelong companions. Masters-prepared Nurse Practitioners have been multiplying rapidly to fill the void left by former general practitioners of medicine. Remember the physician you were brought up with, the person who took the time to ask you how your life was proceeding? He's mostly gone, but a new advocate has arrived in the person of the Nurse Practitioner. Nurses have been formally educated as primary healthcare providers to respond to and treat what is happening in your life. Still fighting for physician-blocked third party reimbursement, they've once again devoted the time necessary to address the concerns of your entire life. Instead of merely treating disease, they evaluate your health. These nurses are less expensive since it's cheaper to preserve what is whole, rather than fixing what is broken. However, if you need a physician, your nurse will help you select the right one. Does everybody need such a nurse in his life? Probably.

• Inevitably, you will face the issue of death — either through your own illness or that of a loved one. Death comes to every living being and that's why nurses have attuned themselves to this very human phenomenon. Nurses are specialists in the grieving process and perform crisis intervention routinely. Nurses will hold your hand throughout a crisis, but they're also doing more: they're future-oriented, inspecting what you do now as a key to what you'll do in the future. If they tell you that they're acting "intuitively," they really mean that their actions are based on conclusions assimilated from a learned knowledge base, repeated experience and current observation. Thus, when a nurse intervenes with a patient, particularly in the crisis of a death situation, her expertise and your current state of being — your holistic self — therapeutically meld at that one point in time. Nurses rarely have any more significant interactions with their patients. With the loss of a loved one or the threat of your own demise, the nurse helps you either make the next step in life or death, or find a reason to go on.

I felt encouraged by charmed rumor the other day because I know it's true: there are still nurses everywhere. The cult of caring permeates every facet of life, and the profession is flourishing. Although many have abandoned white uniforms, discarded the caps of the past and gone native, they are true believers in every sense. You'll find them reviewing medical records in any healthcare setting (Utilization Review Nurses), cutting escalating healthcare costs. Life Flight Nurses are flying around the nation, transporting accident victims to appropriate facilities. They're staffing the schools (School Nurses) from day-care centers to universities. And, they're staffing the workplace (Industrial/Occupational Nurses) to protect the workers. They are everywhere!

Nurses are conducting research at the university level and at the national level with their own arm of the National Institute of Health. Gradually refining their professional data base as scientists, they are finally substantiating all the intuitive care, the art form of centuries of nursing. The single most undervalued healthcare resource, nurses harbor the solution to the enigma of rising healthcare costs in the United States — themselves.

How did the nurses get to be so good and so smart?

When they finish a basic education of two, three or four years, they pass a state licensure examination which enables them to really start learning. There's rarely a financial payoff for the time and money that they spend on further credentials.

After meeting the obligatory years of experience in their particular field, many nurses pursue certification in their nursing specialty. In terms of self-esteem this pursuit can be a risk-taking behavior; the exams are difficult, the anxiety and preparation intense, and changes for success variable. Like the "board-certified physicians," they sit for exams with 40% and 50% flunk rates — just to get certified. I sacrificed the integrity of my nursing units' budgets one year to buy the staff nurses business cards. I wanted the public to know about the excellence expressed by all those letters behind the staffs' names — CCRN (Certification in Critical Care by the American Association of Critical Care Nurses), RNC (Certification in Adult Nursing, Gerontology, Psychiatry and other fields by the American Nurses Association), CEN (Emergency Department Nursing by The Emergency Nurses Association), AORN (Operating Room Nursing), etc. The list is extensive. While nurses in other countries must satisfy similar requirements in order to practice a specialty, American nurses certify just to prove to their peers and themselves that they're that competent. When the exams are passed, nurses are obligated to engage in periodic recertification processes, attending mandated seminars, conferences and tutorials.

Concurrent with all this activity, nurses are returning to school. Graduate programs are thriving. Beyond this, nurses satisfy the dues of multiple professional organizations. The public is currently rewarding nurses' pursuit of further knowledge and credentialing with increased malpractice insurance costs.

The nurses persevere. They carry a little edge in their minds to get them through the tough times: they are the best nurses the world can imagine. It's all for you, America — you are their patient.

I've been lucky enough to be involved in nursing for over twenty years. The best thing about being a nurse is being able to proudly bind my daily identity to this very special group. As a nurse administrator, I used to pride myself in nursing nurses so they could nurse the patients. But I've changed and grown with the profession. Now, I'm a facilitator. I feel that I'm in a position to promote accountability and autonomy in nursing practice and occasionally to implement beneficial change at strategic points along the continuum of nursing practice. I'm a kind of "point man" for the profession, running constructive interference with the system for the nurses I work with. With their permission and by mutual agreement, I handle the structure. They've got other things to worry about — like their patients. If I can help the nurses with the organization in which they work, they'll be free to help their patients and we all will win. When I get up in the morning, I wonder what good things we'll do together today.

While flying through life with this group, I've soared a lot and crashed a bit. I've experienced burnout, that dreadful response to chronic, unmitigated distress, and felt the bite of severe stress. But I've learned to be energized by the stress of my profession. When a nurse tells me that she's "stressed out," I try to help her figure out what she's going to do with the power of that force.

When a European philosopher asked me what Americans could offer the world in the way of the model for the future, I suggested that we are evolving into a people who are comfortable with change. I was thinking of the more dynamic of my nursing peers. Beyond the global stuff, change is the substance of individual lives and helping individuals to accept changes in their minds and bodies is something nurses are very good at. I'm continually optimistic about our nursing mission and its value to humanity — it just needs to be talked about. Historically nurses have worked so hard that the luxury of introspection avoided them. The current abuse of nurses by the healthcare system has made further avoidance impossible. Nurses are critically examining themselves and the society which has not adequately rewarded them. For the first time since I slipped into the profession, nurses are now talking to each other about each other. They have become supportive and appreciative of each other, fed by the strength of their special art and science. Now, whenever I enter upon a group of nurses I can sense the din and hum of a recently empowered group, finally aware of their worth and necessity. Nurses are becoming acutely *unabused.*

Chapter Two

The Present State of Nursing:
Statistics, Economics, Internal Conflicts and Other Obstacles

Nursing care is holistic, that is, the view that care be directed toward a person as whole, not merely focused on a specific disease or injury, and unique in all that whole encompasses. Nurses are responsible for all aspects of patient care, whether it be physical, emotional, psychological, sociological, technical or cultural. Nurses are the coordinators of the healthcare team providing care 24 hours a day, seven days a week, 52 weeks a year. Nurses must be well educated in the anatomy and physiology of the human body and in tune with the emotional and psycho-social aspects of the patients they care for. Nurses must be leaders, advocates and also skilled technicians. They must be compassionate, patient and understanding.

There are many issues facing nursing today and the one that draws the most attention is the cumulative effect of **NURSE ABUSE** — the shortage of registered nurses at the bedside. After all, without the bedside nurse, the profession of nursing would not exist. There would be no reason to have nurse educators, nurse executives or nurse administrators.

The art and practice of bedside nursing is not performed in an air-conditioned office decorated with pastel paintings where a desk provides space for calendars filled with meeting schedules. Yet it is in such offices where the fate of nursing is being determined.

Healthcare has become big business. The cost-containment crunch has been in effect for many years, leading to the birth of Diagnostic Related Groups (DRGs). Cutting corners and "getting by" with the least amount of staff are now the main objectives for administrators and nursing management. No matter what department is cut, nursing is affected. However, nurses have not abandoned their priorities, as patient care continues to remain the main objective. Yet nurses are now expected to care for a larger number of higher acuity (i.e., sicker) patients, that is, patients who are more acutely ill, with less staff, and in a shorter time span for pay that is not comparable to their worth.

Statistically speaking, there are more registered nurses now than ever before, the number having doubled over the past 30 years to a rate exceeding the population growth.

According to the U.S. Department of Labor Bureau Statistics, the projected number of registered nurses for the year 2000 is 2,018,000. However, the current trend includes the startling estimate that, by the year 2000, *there will be one-half as many nurses as needed* (Naylor 1987, p. 1601).

The predicted need for increased nursing personnel is largely a function of the AIDS epidemic, which is having a profound effect on the entire healthcare industry. The majority of people reported to have AIDS are between the ages of 20 and 45. Also, the number of AIDS cases among infants continues to grow. Health officials estimate that at least 1.5 million Americans are carriers of the disease and project that by 1991 there will be nearly 180,000 deaths caused by the AIDS virus. The statistics are staggering. In addition, the disease carries with it, erroneously, the stigma of being a "gay disease", a fact which has caused people with AIDS to be shunned rather than embraced by society. Considering the impact that the AIDS epidemic is having on the healthcare industry, the alarming prediction of a nurse deficit by the year 2000 is undoubtedly under estimated, for we have yet to witness the peak of either the nursing shortage or the AIDS crisis.

There has been much discussion on whether or not a nursing shortage truly exists. With people living longer, the increased number of patients with multi-system failure means a sicker patient population, necessitating a higher nurse-patient ratio. In 1972, hospitals employed 50 nurses per 100 patients (average daily census). By 1986, that number increased to 91 nurses per 100 patients (Aiken, 1987, p. 642). Nurses aides and LPNs were replaced by the versatile RN. In 1968, RNs accounted for 33% of hospitals' total nursing personnel. By 1986, this increased to 58%. Interestingly enough, as Aiken and Mullinix state, "the shortage of hospital nurses exists during the substantial reduction in hospital inpatient capacity nationally. The demand for acute inpatient care in general hospitals has fallen, resulting in 50 million fewer inpatient days in 1986 than 1981 (Aiken, 1987, p. 641). The magic number of beds closed since 1983 is 40,000, with occupancy rates dropping 63.4% in 1986" (Aiken, 1987, p. 642). Despite all of these reductions in beds and occupancy rates, the nursing shortage worsens. But nurses still continue to care by working harder and faster; they still continue to care.

The demand for nurses is indirectly measured by hospitals according to full-time equivalent (FTE) positions of RNs (Aiken, 1987, p. 642). One FTE is equal to 40 hours per week but may be used as one position or divided up as part-time positions. Vacancy rates cannot measure the need for actual bedside nurses, as other factors such as budget constraints and local wage rates are reflected (Aiken, 1987, p. 642). Thus, the need for nurses at a particular facility is determined by its administration according to its budget. Staff nurses have no input in such matters — another facet of **NURSE ABUSE** — and they may even experience a greater deficit in personnel than is estimated by management. Let's face it, it is the nurse who delivers hands-on care to patients, who truly knows what is needed to provide adequate care. And yet she is the last to be consulted, if she is consulted at all.

In hospitals, vacant positions for RNs have doubled since 1985, according to a December 1987 survey which the American Organization of Nurse Executives supported (Curran, 1987, p. 444). *The American Journal of Nursing (AJN)* mailed a survey regarding vacancy rates for RNs to 2,316 randomly selected hospitals nationwide. Forty-four percent of 1000 hospitals responded, providing data in FTEs for the week of December 1, 1986. The average vacancy rate for RN positions was 11%, with more than two-thirds of the vacancies being full-time positions. Seventeen percent reported no vacancies. The lowest vacancy rates were reported in the states of Minnesota, Iowa, Missouri, North and South Dakota, Nebraska and Kansas. In contrast, the Atlantic states of New York, New Jersey and Pennsylvania reported the largest vacancy rates.

Also surveyed was the length of time needed to recruit nurses. The area with the most trouble was critical care. Eighty-seven percent reported great difficulty in recruiting RNs for critical care units (approximately 60 to 90 days.)

In a study conducted by the American Association of Critical Care Nurses (AACN) from January through

April 1988, the vacancy rate for RNs in critical care was 13.8% despite the employment of 194,000 RNs in critical care areas (*AACN News,* 1988, p. 1). It was predicted that "by 1990 a 42 to 90% increase in the number of critical care nurses will be needed to care for the critically ill" (*AACN News.* 1988, p. 1).

Aiken (1987, p. 642) supplies reasons for the current shortage of RNs:

1. Sicker patients — increased acuity requires more care because of discretionary admissions and shorter length of stay.
2. Changing budget constraints on hospitals.
3. Wages.

Because of their versatility, RNs can be considered the "ultimate" employee. As Aiken (1987, p. 643) points out, "When relative wages are low as compared with other workers, it's to the hospital administrations' advantage to employ RNs even if the pay scale is 20 to 30% higher than aides and LPNs, as RNs need less supervision and assume responsibility for a wide range of duties."

One of the most widely publicized facets of **NURSE ABUSE** relates to inadequate financial compensation for nurses. Historically, wages for nurses have lagged behind other occupations predominantly occupied by women (nursing continues to be a primarily female profession). From 1946 to 1966, nurses' wages increased 58% while teachers' increased 100%. In fact, the fluctuations in nursing salaries over the years can be compared to a ride on a roller coaster. For example, in the 1960s, there was great concern over a serious nursing shortage; the institution of Medicare and Medicaid partially accounted for a substantial wage increase for nurses during that era. Later, in 1971, the institution of hospital and price control, state rate setting and cost-containment efforts caused wages to decline for nurses. Again, wages increased approximately 13% annually in 1980 and 1981 in response to the 1979 nursing shortage. By 1984, the RN vacancy rate plummeted to 3.7%. Subsequently, the institution of DRGs caused financial panic in the healthcare industry, resulting in the lack of any substantial wage increase for nurses. In 1985, teachers averaged salaries 19% higher than RNs. And, in 1986, wages for female professionals and technical workers increased 10% while RNs wages increased a mere 4%. These are perfect examples of the short-term, ineffective solutions that have been attempted in order to reduce the severity of the nursing shortages.

The *AJN Guide to Nursing Career Opportunities 1988* reported results of some 1987 surveys of wages and salaries for nurses. The results of the annual University of Texas survey, up to July 1987, reported a starting salary for staff nurses of $20,964 and an averaged maximum salary of $29,088. Starting rates of head nurses were $26,228 with a maximum of $36,444.

In a different survey by Roth Young Personnel Service, reported by *AJN,* staff nurse salaries ranged from a low of $23,000 to a high of $30,900 with the median being $27,000. Head nurse salaries ranging from $31,000 to $42,000 with a median of $35,800. In this survey, the salaries reported were in conjunction with hospital size in which the low rates were from hospitals with less than or equal to 250 beds; median rates were from hospitals with 250-450 beds; and high rates were from hospitals having more than or equal to 450 beds. This study (*"Nurses Again,"* 1988, p. 112) reveals an unexpected decrease in raise percentage of 3.1 from 4.3 from July 1986 to July 1987 for staff nurses. In fact, in some areas, staff nurses' raises were behind the rate of inflation. Maximum rates increased by 4.8%.

Because of the nursing shortage, many efforts are currently being made to recruit and retain RNs mainly by increasing wages. Salaries are rapidly on the rise, especially in the Northeast states. New strategies include offering hourly pay of $2 to $3 higher than standard for nurses who are able to do without benefit packages (health insurance, vacation and sick time). Also, benefit packages are now being offered that include dental insurance, child care facilities, clinical ladders and flexible staffing along with increases in differential pay for the off shifts. And, of course, there is growth in the use of nursing agencies to supplement existing staff. Working for agencies, nurses can make much more money, select their own hours, and in some cases, receive benefits. Agency nursing is beneficial for the individual but can have detrimental effects on the salaries of those nurses employed in the facilities that use them. Hospitals use agencies as a short-term solution for day-to-day staffing to 'get by' until the shortage of nurses is over. This allows them to keep the salaries of their own employees at a lower-than-equitable level. According to an American Hospital Association survey (*"Nurses Again"*, 1987 p.115), hospitals had increased their use of agencies by 31% from December 1986 to April 1987; more nurses had quit their jobs to join such agencies.

Reports conducted by *AJN* in 1987 show regional differences in salaries and indicate that wages are increasing throughout the United States. The lowest salaries were in the South, while the highest were on the West Coast. An interesting fact, highlighted by *AJN*, 1988, was the significant increase in salary for new graduates in Texas from 1986 to 1987 to the tune of approximately $3,000 to $4,000 per year, and for Long Island's new graduates which began at $27,000 per year, a hike of $4,000.

It is not surprising to see such starting salaries as

employers react to the current nursing shortage. However, nurses are still not adequately paid for years of experience. This is where **NURSE ABUSE** is most evident. In fact, wages increase for the early years of employment, peak and then decline.

In comparing nurses' salaries to those of other professionals (such as lawyers and engineers), starting salaries of the three groups begin in the range of $20,000 to $35,000 per year. However, nurses salaries remain stagnant thereafter while significant increases in salary are evident for the other professionals mentioned. In fact, lawyers and engineers make more money within six years of employment than most nurses make after 20 years of experience.

In nursing, professional experience is a highly valued and sought-after attribute. And yet, nurses are not adequately compensated for longevity. An hourly rate for an experienced RN is usually only 50 cents more than the new graduate. Also, colleagues who had 20 years of experience in nursing were averaging approximately only $2.08 more per hour than new graduates. And merely raising salaries of experienced nurses in order to allow new graduates to remain at a "respectably lower level," thereby reducing wage compression, is certainly not enough, nor is it an answer to a chronically deficient wage and salary program.

I recently learned that a self-employed typist charges $15.00 per hour! The average maximum wage for RNs is approximately $7,000 greater than starting salary. These wage statistics illustrate a situation that is deplorable and an insult to nurses, especially considering the depth of knowledge and technical skill required to do the job, not to mention the fact that the balance of life and death often rests in the nurse's hands.

A registered nurse is educated in the complexity of

the human body. Yes, we now have special areas of expertise, but we are also generalists. We are required to understand the function of all body systems (the heart, lungs, kidney, brain, stomach, bowel, liver, bones, muscles, immune system etc.) and how they integrate with one another; we need to know what to look for in the way of signs and symptoms (which are often subtle), and what a certain disease process does to these systems. We learn what interventions are necessary to treat illnesses and we assess each individual's response to such treatment. We learn to interpret the meaning of lab values (blood and body fluid tests), x-rays and other diagnostic procedures. We must know much about pharmacology — the multiple names of medications, the proper dosages, the side-effects or adverse reactions, compatibility with other medications, when and how often to take them, the differing effects of medications as determined by the route of administration (intravenous, intramuscular, oral, subcutaneous). In life-threatening situations, it is the nurse who is there to recognize and respond first by performing basic or advanced cardiac life support. We make independent decisions in the scope of our nursing practice and are quite prepared to do so. We *collaborate* with physicians as professional colleagues; we do not simply "follow orders." In fact, we frequently refer patients to other healthcare specialties — physical therapy, respiratory therapy, social service, dietary, psychiatry, or community health, based upon individualized patient need.

Nurses are aware of their patients' emotional/psychological states; they are sensitive to their individualized responses to illness, to their developing recovery and, in some cases, to their impending death. They are attuned to the patients' and families' ability to cope with illness, and whether or not the family can cope and support their loved one. In critical care units, patients are surrounded

by the "high tech" machinery — respirators, cardiac monitors, IV pumps and invasive monitoring devices — con-
veying vital information regarding the patients' conditions.
It is the nurse who has the technical knowledge to interpret the data and translate it into a meaningful plan of
care. And it is the nurse who meets the "high touch" needs
of the very human presence attached to all that technology
at the bedside.

Nurses are also teachers. Patient teaching is extremely important because it is the patients' knowledge of
their states of health and illness allows them to be active
and responsible participants in their care. Nurses teach
on a wide variety of topics, ranging from changing ostomy
appliances and wound dressings, to explaining adverse reactions to medications and specific signs and symptoms
that warrant immediate medical attention (as with Diabe-
tes Mellitus or heart attack victims).

Nurses are responsible for assisting the patient with
maintenance of personal hygiene, fluid status (intake and
output), nutritional status and mobility (ambulating patients or exercising muscles on patients who are bedridden), and skin integrity.

Everything a nurse does for a patient must be
documented. Documentation using the framework called
"the nursing process" is unique to nursing, and distinctly
different from the medical model of documentation. It
consists of nursing diagnosis of patient problem, patient
assessment, plan of nursing care, nursing interventions
and evaluation of outcomes of care rendered. The nursing
process is generally recorded in the narrative nurses notes,
where specific patient problems are addressed. Routine
care (such as bathing, turning, ambulation etc.) is usually
recorded on a flowsheet in a check-list format. There are
other forms of required documentation, including frequent
observation sheets, skin integrity sheets, medication

sheets and special procedure sheets. Clearly then, nursing involves much paperwork, and this is a frequently voiced complaint of many caregivers, who feel torn by the amount of time they *can't* spend at the bedside. Unfortunately, the nurse is forced to work with the knowledge that failing to chart translates into failing to render care — "if it wasn't charted, it wasn't done."

Ethical dilemmas arise frequently in nursing. The DNR (do not resuscitate) order is a case in point: it can only be written by a physician in circumstances where there is no medical treatment that would change the patient's condition (as with terminal cancer or end-stage organ disease). Many factors affect this issue, the major one being patient competency. However, the family is always consulted before a decision is made. Most often, the patient is the one to request that no "heroics" be done to prolong his or her life. But it is usually the family that refuses to accept the death of a loved one and will not authorize a DNR status. Thus, the nurse gets caught in the middle — she knows the patient's wishes were not to be resuscitated, but she is confronted with a family that cannot accept the inevitability of their loved one's death. There is nothing worse than performing CPR, and watching all the invasive procedures that go with it, on a person who requested otherwise. Often, these patients are on nursing units for long periods of time and nurses grow to care about and respect them in a profound way. There can be no gray area in these cases. "Slow codes" are not the answer; either you resuscitate or you don't. Unfortunately, all too frequently, we *do* when we *shouldn't*.

With increased responsibility comes the need for additional continuing education. Nursing and medical interventions change constantly, so nurses must keep abreast of the latest developments. Continuing education is mandatory for nursing licensure, but most nurses go far beyond what is required to improve their practice. There is never too much to learn in healthcare and being a nurse includes a career-long commitment to continuing education. With increased responsibility goes increased accountability, a fact which is borne out by the importance of each nurse carrying independent malpractice insurance. We are liable for what we do, and susceptible to being cited in lawsuits.

Considering the multifaceted demands, stressors, and responsibilities which exist in the nursing profession today, coupled with the inequitable monetary compensation nurses receive for shouldering such a burden, it stands to reason that women in the work force are choosing other careers. Far more lucrative and prestigious options are available to women of the '90s, and nursing is losing ground in recruitment.

Supply and Demand

The demand for RNs has risen dramatically, the same time enrollment in nursing schools has plummeted. Since 1983, nursing school enrollments have fallen off by 20% (Aiken, 1987, p. 644).

Cooperative Institutional Research Program (CIRP) surveyed almost 300,000 college freshmen at nearly 600 institutions in the fall of 1986. A follow-up survey of freshmen who began four-year nursing degrees in the fall of 1982 showed that 52.4% changed their major. In two-year programs, 14.6% did the same (Green, 1987, p. 1610).

In the fall of 1986, 20,000 freshmen women planned to become nurses compared to 43,000 in the fall of 1983. The annual number of new graduates is predicted to drop from a high of 82,700 in 1985 to 68,700 or less by 1995 (Aiken, 1987, p. 644). All types of RN programs have had a decrease in enrollments as a result of the declining interest in nursing as a career choice. The University of California-Los Angeles reported a 50% decrease since 1974 of women interested in pursuing a nursing career, as opposed to an almost three-fold increase among those interested in business. Thirty five percent of newly practicing physicians are women; 40% of new entrants in law schools and the majority of new entrants in accounting are women as well.

In 1984, 8.3% of freshman women were aspiring nurses. By 1986, that number decreased to 5.1% (Green, 1987, p. 1610). Many women are choosing to become physicians instead of nurses because they now have such an option. As Green (Green, 1987, p. 1612) stated:

"By 1990 or 1991 American colleges will award some 14,500 BSN degrees compared to almost 16,000 MD degrees (to women). The last numbers are truly startling and place the much discussed physician surplus/nursing shortage in a very interesting and very different perspective".

CIRP data date back 21 years, and it reveals significant changes in attitudes, values, educational achievements and life goals of college students in America. It appears that the '80s freshmen are "yuppie" types. In fact, the survey dated has shown a transition of life goals from "developing a meaningful philosophy of life," stated by college students in the late 60s, to "being very well-off financially." The transition is evident in the shift away from traditional careers. College freshmen now seem to be more materialistic and interested in striving to obtain high-paying, high-status jobs, turning away from altruistic careers such as nursing, teaching and social service.

If becoming "very well-off financially" is the priority in choosing a career path, then a job in healthcare (including respiratory or physical therapy, social work, lab or medical technology, nursing etc.) or teaching is not appropriate because large financial rewards are unlikely. A different reward exists in careers that focus on helping others — one that may come simply by knowing that your expertise has made a difference in another person's life. Perhaps one of the most blatant manifestations of **NURSE ABUSE** is the pervasiveness of roadblocks that prevent nurses from accomplishing all that they are capable of, depriving them of the personal reward and self-fulfillment that is their due.

Good Old Uncle Sam

Education is costly today and future monetary gains just do not add up if one pursues a nursing career. The practical answer to that problem is financial support for aspiring nurses. The Reagan Administration tried to completely cut off any federal funding for nursing education already allocated through previous legislation. This was apparently the result of reports conducted earlier by the Department of Health and Human Services (DHHS). For example, in 1986 the American Hospital Association (AHA) was reporting that high vacancy rates in nursing positions were disruptive to patient care, while the DHHS concluded that the national supply of nurses was in balance with the current demand (Aiken, 1987, p. 1642). Despite conflicting documentation from other sources which clearly stated that, indeed, there was a shortage of nurses, the DHHS continued to state that educational support should be eliminated (another prime example of **NURSE ABUSE**). Attempts at eliminating federal funding for nursing were thwarted by Congress.

But some legislators are taking the initiative in discussing the nursing shortage and developing ways to actively study and support nursing issues. Congress has initiated legislation through the Senate Labor and Human Resources committee that would authorize allocation of $5 million to study and fund projects to alleviate the problem (Nursing Shortage Reduction Act of 1987, S.1402) which was proposed in 1987 (Inglehart, 1987, p. 650). In 1988, Congress reauthorized the Nurse Education Act, now part of the Omnibus Health Bill, providing $80 million in 1989 (the most money authorized since 1981), $106 million in 1990 and $123 million in 1991 for nursing education. Such federal spending has had its peaks and valleys in the past. The peak of allocated monies for nursing-related purposes, in 1973, amounted to $160.6 million and concentrated on supporting nursing schools and students. Each year since, the amount of federal spending has decreased to a low of $48.5 million in 1983.

Many legislative acts are targeted at relieving the nursing shortage. In October of 1988, the Senate and the House of Representatives approved a bill that supports nursing education, nurse recruitment centers, innovative practice models and other programs. Millions of dollars are now proposed for provisions such as long-term care nursing models, nursing practice models, nurses as patient care managers, management structures, career progression strategies for RNs, innovative payment structures and improved working conditions, Medicare support for nurse clinical training and even direct reimbursement for certain Medicare services (Harrington, 1988, p. 119). These topics are included in different legislative bills and committees, and show the general direction the government is taking with respect to the nursing shortage dilemma. Nevertheless, this "support" by the government is not so much a vote of confidence in the nursing *profession* as it is a response to a national *crisis* known as the nursing shortage. As seen in the past, there is no guarantee that in years to come these strategies and measures will not be reduced or eliminated as soon as the "shortage" is "cured."

Nursing organizations have learned to play the political "game" through lobbying for and against policies that directly affect the profession on the national level. Each organization has its own priorities, but a common goal is one of improving nursing's political position through solidarity (Burda, 1987, p. 28). The No.1 priority has been to receive direct reimbursement for nursing services. Currently, nurses are paid by their employers. There is no separate fee for nursing services charged to insurance companies, Medicare or patients directly. The cost of nursing services is factored into the sum of charges that includes the cost of the room, food and miscellaneous supplies (bandages, razors, needles, syringes etc.). This is the major cause of wage compression for nurses, as the employer controls the hourly rate or salary of its employees according to the yearly budget constraints. Direct reimbursement for nursing service would completely change the current practice of payment for nurses. In other words, the employer would lose control over wages for nurses and would receive less money from those who pay the bills. This brings fierce opposition from hospital organizations and physicians. Physicians are directly reimbursed from insurance companies for their service. Thus, if nursing becomes financially independent through direct reimbursement, physicians and employers feel it will significantly cut into their "piece of the pie." But financial reimbursement means autonomy for nurses and that is where some of the most heated battles are being fought today. It is obvious that all nurses have to get politically active to ensure meaningful and long-lasting changes in the profession.

Internal Conflicts

Internal conflicts in the nursing community have stymied progress on political and professional issues. The major issues causing conflict today revolve around the definition of what constitutes a professional and appropriate entry level into practice. The question, "Is nursing a profession?" has been asked frequently in recent years. Most nurses say "yes," regardless of their basic level of entry into practice. Nursing leaders and organizations have attempted to standardized educational preparation by having the entry-level into practice be the baccalaureate degree (BSN).

There are now three educational preparations for registered nurses: the two-year associate degree program, the three-year diploma program and the four-year baccalaureate degree program. However, professions in medicine and law basically follow one educational program.

In striving to have nursing recognized as a bona fide profession, the ANA approved a policy that categorizes nurses into two groups: "professional nurse" and "technical nurse." The minimum educational requirement for the "professional nurse" would be the baccalaureate degree while the associate degree, program defines the "technical" category. All RNs presently licensed would be "grand-fathered" into their respective categories. The institution of this plan has to be initiated by individual states, and each state organization is working to bring this about, some more rapidly than others. North Dakota standardized its educational preparations by requiring curricula for LPNs to enter associate degree programs and for RNs to enter baccalaureate degree programs (Inglehart, 1987, p. 649). This action is occurring in many states. The Massachusetts Nurses Association developed a bill in November of 1987 for the "RN professional" and "RN associate." Currently practicing LPNs and RNs without a BSN would be "grandfathered" into the "associate" category and RNs with a BSN or more would be placed in the 'professional' category. Other states which may soon follow this lead include Wisconsin, Illinois, Maine, Minnesota and Texas. Of course, the suggestion of all nursing organizations is to encourage all nurses presently licensed to achieve higher education in BSN programs, and for LPNs to work toward an RN degree.

A point of interest for nurses is how the courts view nursing with regard to professional status. Factors indicative of professionalism in a court of law include a code of ethics, a strong research program, authority and prestige associated with the field, altruism and, most importantly, consistent, systematic educational requirements (Segal, 1985, p. 43). Such educational requirements are considered necessary in weeding out those not qualified or not committed to the field, insuring specialized knowledge and separating non-professionals in related fields. Thus, the treatment of physicians and nurses in lawsuits differs because, in the view of the courts, their curricula are different. Nurses are "trained" and doctors are "educated."

The statute of limitations requires a lawsuit to be filed within a reasonable period of time after the alleged act has transpired. Because of the growing volume of malpractice suits, many state legislatures have decreased the time period required in order to lessen the burden on the courts. The statute of limitations for ordinary negligence (the category which applies to nurses) is approximately two years, whereas professional negligence has been shortened to about one year. This distinction favors the professional. Not that negligence or malpractice should be waived in any case, but this distinction contributes to the image of inferiority held by the courts and the public with respect to nurses.

The AMA's "Believe It Or Not"

Despite the feeling that it's the ninth inning with two outs for the trailing home team, nursing has been taking its time to resolve its own conflicts and find solutions to the shortage and the entry-level question, while the American Medical Association (AMA) has been planning its own strategy in the dugout. The AMA has picked up on the two biggest issues in nursing today, professionalism and the shortage, and proposed its own solution by inventing yet another "bedside caregiver" called the registered care technologist (RCT). Two types of RCT have been proposed by the AMA: basic and advanced. The educational requirement for the basic RCT would be nine months of training, with responsibilities to include monitoring of vital signs, intake and output; bathing, feeding and ambulating patients; observing and recording certain assessment findings, and monitoring responses to routine medications. The advanced RCT training would last 18 months and would qualify the practitioner to monitor patients receiving IV therapy, TPN, mechanical ventilation, cardiac monitoring and CVP lines in critical care units (Schull, 1988, p. 28).

The pursuit of more autonomy in nursing by attempting to increase educational requirements for entry level into nursing practice has caused the AMA to conclude that further education takes nurses away from the bedside. The shortage only serves to validate that thinking.

It is obvious that many physicians continue to have a simplistic view of what nursing is all about. For example, bathing a patient may seem only a basic, uncomplicated *task*, but it can incorporate the unique, finely tuned *skill* of nursing assessment. Nurses can pick up physical clues on every body system by keen observation and discriminating touch, and can obtain information on the patients' emotional and psychological states as well.

The unrealistic aspect of this proposal is the idea that RCTs will be supervised by the physicians themselves. Nurses anticipate that they themselves would end up with this responsibility, as few physicians are available seven days a week to keep abreast on such "technical" aspects of patient care. To add insult to injury, the AMA suggests that "nurses with 'sufficient experience at the bedside' could get RCT licenses ... and advanced certification 'will be available for current RNs who wish to remain at the bedside" (Service, 1988, p. 7). Professional nurses are understandably outraged by such a proposal. It is one more example of how little value is placed on the extensive knowledge and experience of the registered professional nurse — it is one more example of **NURSE ABUSE**. Fortunately, thanks largely to a unified demonstration of *strong* opposition to this proposal by over 100 nursing, healthcare and consumer organizations around the country, this proposal was abandoned by the AMA after its House of Delegates voted on June 28, 1990 to halt further recruitment and training efforts.

Another implication of this proposal included competition for federal funding between nursing-related issues and RCT education. And let us not forget wage rates for RCTs in relation to nurses: There have finally been some significant, long-overdue increases in wages for nurses. Competing wage rates for RCTs could have halted all present and future progress, and caused further compression of wages for nurses.

The AMA did not consult the ANA in developing this proposal, apparently believing that it is not a nursing issue. How a proposed solution to the shortage of nurses could ignore nursing is beyond this nurse! Evidently, the AMA has forgotten the cardinal rule in healthcare: teamwork wins the game. No matter how you cut it, there *is* a nursing shortage. Filling the gaps with anything but nurses is far from a solution.

The View Of The Expert Witness: The Nurse

How do nurses feel about the current state of nursing? How has the shortage affected them? Some national nursing journals have sought the answers to those questions by polling their subscribers and publishing their responses.

In July 1987, *Nursing87* polled its subscribers regarding the effects of the nursing shortage. A separate survey was also sent to 500 nurses in nursing management (also called nurse executives), the majority being directors of Nursing (DONs). Results of the two surveys were compared to determine if the effects of the shortage were the same for both groups. Specific areas covered in the survey included, "current hiring, staffing and retention practices; nurses' mobility and job satisfaction; nurses' thoughts on the future of the profession; whether they'd recommend nursing as a career "("Nursing Shortage", 1988, p. 33).

The two groups surveyed were concerned with the shortage: 47% of the nurse readers were "moderately concerned," while 64% of the nurse executives were "concerned." Most respondents stated that the hospitals they were affiliated with were having difficulty hiring and retaining RNs; nurse executives agreed. Both recognized new hiring practices were being instituted in their facilities. Fifty one percent reported the hiring of new graduates for critical care areas; 48% noted the use of agency nurses to fill staffing gaps; 30% noted increased use of LPNs; 28% noted increases in the use of nursing assistants.

A change in hiring patterns emerged, as evidenced by 72% of nurse readers and 67% of nurse executives responding that their hospitals had not given priority to hiring baccalaureate-prepared nurses. One-third of those hospitals surveyed had previously given priority to nurses prepared at the baccalaureate level. Some respondents also stated that differentials for having a BSN were disappearing. As a result, staffing patterns had also changed dramatically, including increased use of overtime, shift rotation and weekend assignments.

An interesting discrepancy between the two groups appeared in response to increases in salary and benefits. Fifty nine percent of the nurses polled reported no increase in pay or benefits at that time, whereas 58% of the nurse executives reported a pay increase in response to the nursing shortage and 24% reported an increase in benefits. As *Nursing88* pointed out, the nurse executives may have been referring to increased starting rates for new recruits, or to policies "in the works," but not yet enacted. Still, the nurses polled were not yet aware of these financial gains and, as stated previously, the percentage of wage increases in 1987 was small and less than the year before. Significantly, many nurse executives were concerned that increases in salaries for RNs, though limited these increases may be, might discourage the hiring of as many RNs by their CEOs. This practice of offering an improvement in one area at the expense of another — in this case, increased salary at the expense of staffing — is another classic example of **NURSE ABUSE.**

Staff nurses and nursing management apparently are not discussing the shortage. Only 32% of the nurses stated that their directors of nursing discussed the immediate and future implications of the shortage and what was to be done about it in their respective facilities. In contrast, 84% of the nurse executives stated they did otherwise.

When asked if doctors were aware of the nursing shortage, 87% of the nurse executives and 51% of the nurse respondents said yes; 35% didn't know. Regarding administrator's priorities in the wake of this shortage, 51% of nurse executives stated that their CEOs were giving the shortage "high" priority and 39% reported "medium" priority. Most nurses (69%) felt that the public was aware of the problem and 80% of the nurses said that their friends were interested enough to discuss it with them.

With regard to job satisfaction, the nurses polled were asked to rate their jobs on a scale of 1 to 5, 1 being very dissatisfied and 5 being very satisfied. Overall, the majority was near the middle, giving a 3.1 as an average rating. Nine percent were very satisfied and 9% were very dissatisfied. The "very satisfied" nurses were noted to be working in facilities with better staffing, where they were less likely to report hiring and retention difficulties. They also worked in facilities that reported increases in salaries and benefits, and practiced primary nursing. In addition, they were less likely to report an increase in overtime, shift rotation or weekend assignments. Another interesting characteristic of this group is that it was not comprised of staff nurses; the job title reported was listed under "other" (meaning nurse coordinator, educator, clinician, clinical specialist and so on, or as assistant director of nursing) ("Nursing Shortage", 1988, p. 33).

When asked what they would do if the opportunity arose to choose nursing again as their career, 31% would, 35% might and 33% would not. Thirty eight percent had encouraged others to become nurses while 60% had not.

As expected, of the "very satisfied" respondents, 59% were more willing to choose nursing again, while 15% would not, and 35% of them had not encouraged others to follow a career path in nursing.

Job turnover was also surveyed and, not surprisingly, 55% had changed jobs within the past five years. Thirty percent had changed jobs once, 15% twice and 10%

three or more times. The average stay for a nurse in one job was seven years, and 61% had stated that they hadn't stayed long enough to be vested for retirement.

Reasons for "job hopping" included:

- move/change in spouse's job
- better staffing/more manageable work load/less stress
- better salary/benefits
- more autonomy
- professional growth and development/more challenge
- change of field
- better hours, working conditions, flexibility and so on ("Nursing Shortage", 1988, p. 33)

The editors of *Nursing87* received responses on more issues than they had originally intended. Apparently, many nurses viewed the poll as an opportunity to speak their minds about a variety of critical nursing issues. The editors of *Nursing87* noticed that, and felt obligated to print what was on the minds of those nurses.

The perils of short staffing was one of the many issues brought up. Higher patient acuity without a corresponding increase in staffing is a recipe for dangerous clinical situations and the compromised relationship which results — as many nurses reported. This article makes it very clear that nurses are working more overtime, including double shifts. Part-timers are practically working full-time, and full-timers are adding more and more time to their weekly commitments. New grads are being "baptized by fire," with increased responsibilities exceeding their current competency level, leading them to certain frustration and eventual burnout. This situation causes increased stress on existing, experienced staff members, who feel they can't rely on their new colleagues. Again, this leads to increased fear, apprehension and more burnout.

Others reported frustration at the declining emphasis on patient teaching, as nurses must go from task to task, just to get their work done. These nurses (and all nurses) are concerned with giving good care. Nursing is not factory work on inanimate objects. It is "people work" which deals with the vicissitudes of human life. Many nurses are leaving their eight - 10- and 12- hour work days feeling exhausted and, in some cases, physically ill, as they've often found themselves having to work through breaks and lunches. It's almost impossible to find time for such important interventions such as holding the hand of a dying patient to lend comfort, or spending time with the family of a young trauma victim who is not expected to survive, or teaching a first-time mother what she needs to know before discharge (now sometimes less than 24 hours after admission).

The basic physical tasks must be completed, and it seems as though all of the nurse's time is tied up in just that — the completion of *tasks,* and not the provision of quality *care* which nurses are educated to impart. Nurses are not there simply to give baths, feed people and dole out medication. Again, nursing care is holistic in scope, and resorting to the archaic practice of task-oriented nursing is unacceptable. The inability of nurses to live up to their own high standards of care is extremely difficult for them to tolerate, and is causing them increasing distress.

Resentment toward nursing management and administration was quite evident in this poll. There proved to be a wall between staff nurses and administrators that continues to grow rapidly as time goes on. Lack of input by staff nurses on issues that directly affect nursing care is an aspect of **NURSE ABUSE** that infuriates nurses everywhere. The majority of complaints were aimed at nursing management, for its lack of support. Many nurses wondered if these managers remembered their "roots," or if they had been in their offices too long. One nurse described a typical scenario that has plagued nursing since its inception.

> "The nurses in our obstetric floor had been complaining for a long time to their DON and director of personnel that they were working under dangerous conditions and were too short-staffed. Management kept telling them, 'it's not in the budget to hire. Sorry.' The doctors finally got together and complained to the president of the hospital, saying they'd pull out if there weren't enough nurses. Needless to say, jobs opened up and RN's were hired! But we still don't have a voice" ("Nursing Shortage", 1988, p. 33).

Others responded: "Our DON says, 'if you're so unhappy with your job, just quit.' Is that support or what?" ("Nursing Shortage", 1988, p. 33.), and

> "How is it that nursing allowed its staffing to be cut at a time when patients were sicker than ever? I blame that on poor nursing leadership nationwide. These nurses with their PhD's and Masters and clinical specialties sit in their ivory towers and preach about how we should 'work smarter, not harder,' and that doesn't help those of us on the front lines at all. They have no idea what we go through day by day just trying to get the work done. And if you complain or try to suggest changes, they label you a troublemaker" ("Nursing Shortage", 1988, p. 33).

This is particularly distressing because the only

people who seem to truly understand such critical nursing issues are other nurses, and if staff nurses can not turn to their nursing leaders for support, then who can they turn to? This ignites yet another internal conflict that plagues nursing. We fight among ourselves out of frustration, and because we lack control over our own practice. Staff nurses are truly feeling the crunch when it comes to the quality of patient care, and nursing managers are feeling the crunch from their superiors. As a result, they fail to support their staffs, for fear of losing their jobs.

The question of the proposed entry level for nursing was a sore point for diploma nurses in this survey. They felt put down for not having a degree, and undervalued for the knowledge and skill they possess. The baccalaureate-degree nurses felt let down for their under-appreciated hard work, and for the additional expense to completing a higher education (that does not pay off). They felt criti-cized for not having enough clinical experience by their non-degree peers, as well. As stated by one nurse, "a BSN degree does not a nurse make ... " ("Nursing Shortage", 1988, p. 33.).

But does a collegiate diploma make a nurse? Every nurse is green when she or he first comes out of school. *Experience* makes a nurse, and it's up to each individual to educate himself or herself to become the best nurse pos-sible. This bickering among ourselves serves no purpose, and hinders the progress that nursing must make.

What nurses in this poll ("Nursing Shortage", 1988, p. 33) wanted the most in evaluating their jobs in order of priority include factors such as sufficient nursing staff, support from nursing management, minimum of every other weekend off, support from administration, perma-nent shift assignment, benefits, salary, staffing patterns in general, support from doctors, opportunity in advancement, location and staff development. Of course, wages were a factor. Many nurses feel perpetually underpaid, never being recognized financially for their worth. One nurse summed it up well. "The hours and pay stink. Some days I say, 'why me' ... I could work as a grocery clerk ... I almost have a PhD and make less than others graduating with a BS in another field ... if we were men, our salary would be three times what it is now, with less work."

Research has compared earnings of women with men and of minorities (men and women) with white men. Carlson (1988, p. 530) compared the earnings of women and ethnic minorities with white men. Overall, the earnings gap decreased throughout the years studied for all groups except for white women "whose mean earnings relative to white men's changed little between 1969 and 1979." However, it was noted that all women consistently earned substantially less than minority and white men. And "unmeasured influences on earnings, including discrimination, affected women more than men" (Carlson, 1988, p. 544). White and Puerto Rican women were the only groups of women that failed to gain in relation to white men. One explanation for the stagnation of earnings for white women was the dramatic increase in labor market participation by white women in the 1970s; thus, the average work experience of those women was lower than that of white men (Carlson, 1988, p.45). However, all other groups "gained in earnings relative to white men despite their having also increased their labor market participation" (Carlson, 1988, p. 45). In a study conducted by Blau and Beller (1988) comparing earnings differentials by gender, the earnings of women compared to men proved better in the 1970s than previously estimated. In short, they adjusted time inputs (hours and weeks worked) and wages differently, and came up with higher earnings percentages for women in the male-female ratio for the periods between 1971 and 1981. Blau and Beller (1988) concluded that the

Equal Employment Opportunity laws, changes in women's aspirations and improved qualifications contributed to the narrowed earnings gap. However, the facts indicate that the extent of gain for white women steadily declines with age and is uniform for black women (Blau and Beller, 1988, p. 524). And, it was stated that "previous research suggests that, all else equal, predominantly male occupations and integrated occupations pay more than predominantly female occupations" (Blau and Beller, 1988, p. 518). Finally, in a survey to ascertain sex biases in comparable-worth analysis, it was found that "jobs were perceived as requiring relatively more persuasive ability, (and) were rated as relatively higher in overall monetary worth when they were performed by a male incumbent, rather than by a female."

It is encouraging to see a narrowing earnings gap between men and women but a significant gap still exists — that is a fact. And that fact is difficult to understand and accept on the threshold of the 21st century. **NURSE ABUSE** stems from the fact that women are an oppressed group, and they continue to be discriminated against in terms of monetary gain for comparable worth. The nursing profession is predominantly made up of women; therefore, nurses are abused as a matter of course.

The editors of *Nursing88* compared results of their 1987 job satisfaction poll to a similar poll they conducted in 1978. It was noted that 79% of the respondents in 1978 were moderately or very satisfied with their jobs, while only 34% of the respondents felt this way less than a decade later. Even more significant, in 1978, 31% were very satisfied, compared to a mere 9% in the 1987 poll.

As concluded by the editors of *Nursing88,* the critical issue was simply this:

"Nurses still care deeply about their patients ... these nurses are keeping patients alive every day. Theircontributions go unheralded, but the healthcare system would be lost without them. If nursing isn't going to lost its best and brightest, nursing leaders have to be more realistic about enormous needs of patients, more responsive to the needs of nurses and more politically assertive inside and outside the workplace. Yes, America needs nurses — and they're worth fighting for" (Nursing Shortage, 1988, p. 33).

The American Journal of Nursing (AJN) did a survey in June 1987 entitled "What Keeps Nurses in Nursing." Results were reported in the February 1988 edition. The poll was targeted at staff nurses, head nurses, and assistant head nurses to obtain feedback on what "bedside nurses want and need to stay in practice" (Hartley and Huey, 1988, p. 181).

Some interesting differences emerged in what these respondents felt was important with respect to their jobs and benefits. The survey categorized the respondents as "leavers" (within three years) and "stayers" (will stay in nursing at least three more years). An initially encouraging result was that 3 to ten nurses would stay in nursing at least three more years. However, sadly, many of those nurses stay in the profession because they feel "trapped," and are unhappy with nursing. In fact, those who were unhappy would not encourage others to pursue a career in the nursing profession.

Both groups in Hartley and Huey's (1988) article agreed on the 10 most important factors which include competent RN staff; the freedom to exercise nursing judgment for patient care; adequate RN to patient ratio; support from nurse administrators; available help when a patient needs extra care; a sense of being an important member of the healthcare team; positive interactions with other nurses; adequate salary; desired work schedule available; and up-to-date nursing and medical procedures. The 10 dissatisfying factors included availability of child care facilities; support from hospital administrators; amount of paperwork; support from nurse administrators; salary, availability of help when a patient needs extra care — RN to patient ratio; availability of continuing education opportunities; availability of inservice education and fringe benefits.

Two new areas of dissatisfaction for nurses today include the nurse-patient ratio and the availability of additional staff when patient needs warrant it. A frequent response from the nurses in this 1987 poll cited their inability to meet their own expectations in giving the kind of care they assessed for their patients. Other frustrations pointed to non-nursing duties, increased paperwork, nurse-patient ratio with increased patient acuity, salary, lack of support from nursing management and administration, and lack of input in nursing-related matters.

Support from administration, or lack thereof, has a direct effect on job satisfaction for nurses. Unfortunately, in both surveys, the majority felt abandoned by their administrators. One nurse with over 10 years' experience responded to the *AJN* survey by stating:

> "The emphasis is no longer on quality care. Nurses would probably put up with less-than-fabulous salaries (we already do), but administrators are not in touch enough with what their employees do to provide an environment that would satisfy nurses far more than dollars would" (Hartley and Huey, 1988, p. 186).

Another nurse proves that point by stating:

"I have recently changed jobs from an employer who devalued nurses to one who placed great value on individual care. The emphasis has gone from saving money at the cost of quality to one of quality care with caution towards costs. I am much happier now" (Hartley and Huey, 1988, p. 187).

Thus the major issues — inadequate staffing, low wages, poor communication, increased demands due to paperwork, decline in patient contact, poor leadership and lack of unity in the profession.

Researchers suggested that nursing leaders better communicate with their nurses, work with them to fulfill their needs. Today, however, events such as expanding bed capacity on nursing units where staffing has already been communicated as being at a dangerous level, evokes the patronizing response from administrators of "we hear ya." But actions are few and far between as the pool of nurses shrinks.

A key statement was made in an article published by *RN Magazine;*

" ... the drain will continue until people who run hospitals begin to understand that nurses really are dedicated professionals and not just an anonymous mass of bodies to be shuffled into so many slots. Rigid authoritarianism may have worked 50 years ago, but modern administrators have got to realize that nurses don't have to put up with it anymore. They have too many alternatives they can take" ("Getting Fed Up", 1981, p. 18).

These problems must be addressed and resolved in ways

that contribute to a progressive increase in the status of nursing, both within the healthcare arena and society at large. The lack of effective leadership and unity among nurses inhibits nursing's progress from year to year. It stands to reason that if nurses were satisfied with working conditions and feel they are communicating with administrators, there would be less turnover, better morale and concomitant cost containment. Why can't administrators recognize this fact and act on it? What are they afraid of? One possible answer appears self evident: loss of control. Nurses are overworked, underpaid, underappreciated, overstressed and ultimately fed up with being treated like children. **NURSE ABUSE** must cease, for it has caused a crisis in the profession of nursing in particular, and the healthcare system in general. The nursing shortage is certain to get progressively worse before it gets better, as nursing school enrollments have fallen short of the ever-increasing demand. Radical change is required *now*, before things get even worse.

The typical staff nurse is routinely inundated with non-nursing duties that waste precious time — taking specimens to the lab; picking up medication from the pharmacy; moving and washing beds; mopping up spills on the off-shifts; hiding linen the day before a holiday because the laundry staff may not work holidays; putting charts together and answering a phone that rings continuously because there is no unit secretary available (for a variety of reasons); emptying the overflowing garbage barrels; taking lab or procedure results over the phone due to the lack of "state-of-the-art" computer systems; and more.

All these tasks because those responsible for such duties are "too busy," "short-staffed" or simply "not budgeted for," as is so commonly the case on the evening and night shifts. So who picks up the slack? Nursing! And you can bet that hospital administrators rely on this fact.

With regard to non-nursing duties, we are our own worst enemies *because we do them.*

On a personal note, I believe that the majority of nurses do enjoy their jobs when given the opportunity to practice nursing as they know it should be practiced. Why else would they be hanging on? But, they are "hanging on" by a thread, waiting for a light at the end of the tunnel. That source of light must come from within. As stated previously, there are more registered professional nurses working now than ever before. The time has come to prove that there is power in numbers. As a staff nurse, these issues truly hit home for me. I enjoy being a nurse, and I am proud to say so. For me, nursing is a challenging, compassionate, exciting career, essential for the mainte-nance of health. Nurses are the backbone of healthcare, and account for the largest number of healthcare providers in the industry. Without us, there is no healthcare indus-try. We must recognize our strength and stand together, before we allow others to do with us what they will. We must take control of our own destinies. We must refuse to be intimidated by autocratic management tactics by say-ing "No" to unsafe work assignments, inadequate wages, intolerable working conditions and a lack of respect and support from our nursing leaders, other healthcare profes-sionals, government officials and the public.

The nursing shortages of the past and present are not the problem. Rather they are among the symptoms — the symptoms of **NURSE ABUSE**.

We must treat **NURSE ABUSE** as a disease and eradicate it from our profession. We have the ability to do it by speaking out and standing up for what we believe in nursing. Only then will nursing be healthy enough to re-cruit and retain its best and brightest.

References

Aiken, L.H., & Mullinix, C.F. (1987). The nursing shortage: Myth or reality. *New England Journal of Medicine, 217*(10).

AJN guide nursing career opportunities. (1988).
New York: American Journal of Nursing Co.

Blau, F.D., & Beller, A.H. (1988). Trends in earnings differentials by gender, 1971-1981. *Industrial and Labor
Relations Review, 41*(4).

Burda, K. (1987). Nursing lobby exerting new found
power in Washington. *Modern Health Care, 12.*

Carlson, L.A., & Swartz, C. (1988). The earnings of
women and ethnic minorities, 1959-1979. *Industrial
and Labor Relations Review, 41*(4).

Curran, C.R., Minnick, A., & Moss, J. (1987). Who needs
nurses? *American Journal of Nursing, 87*(4).

Getting fed up? (1981). *RN, 44*(1).

Green, K. (1987). What the freshmen tell us. Nurses for
the future: A special supplement. *American Journal of
Nursing,* December; *87*(12).

Harrington, C. (1988). A policy agenda for the nursing shortage. *Nursing Outlook,* May/June. *36*(3).

Hartley, S., & Huey, F.L. (1988). What keeps nurses in nursing, 3,500 nurses tell their stories. *American Journal of Nursing*, *88*(2).

Inglehart, J.K. (1987). Health Policy Report. Problems facing the nursing profession. *New England Journal of Medicine,* September 3; *217*(10); p. 650.

Landmark study confirms nursing shortage problem. (1988). *AACN News,* August.

McArthur, L.Z., & Obrant, S.W. (1986). Sex biases in comparable worth analysis. Journal of *Applied Social Psychology, 16*(9).

Naylor, MD, & Sherman, M.B. (1987). Nurses for the future; wanted: The best and brightest. *American Journal of Nursing, (12)*: 1601.

Nurses again lost some economic ground in '87. (1988). *American Journal of Nursing, 88*(1): 112.

Nursing shortage poll report. (1988). *Nursing 88, 18*(2).

Schull, P.D. (1988). The AMA solution-another warning for nursing. *Nursing88, 18*(7).

Segal, E.T. (1985). Is nursing a profession? *Nursing 85, 15*(6).

Service, R. (1988). An alarming proposal. Editorial. *RN, 6.*

Chapter Three

Forms of Nurse Abuse

It's 11 p.m. You are the charge nurse for the midnight to 8 a.m. shift in a 10-bed medical-surgical intensive care Unit (ICU). Conscientious, you always arrive "just a few minutes early" for your shift. You leave the locker room after depositing your belongings and head for the unit. As you walk to the nurse's station through the electric doors, you note the area is astir with activity.

Right on your heels is a patient being transferred to the intensive care unit (ICU) from the emergency room. A "code blue", or patient having a cardiac arrest, is taking place in bed 7. The phone is ringing off the hook ... the laboratory calling with blood analysis results, the admitting office calling to find out the correct patient census, the family of the patient who has just been admitted to the unit calling to find out his status. More and more frequently, the scenario being played out before your eyes is the norm for your shift. The charge nurse from the previous shift is tugging at your arm, ready to start report, albeit 15 minutes early, because she has "had enough" and wants to go home on time. She tells you that there were supposed to be four nurses booked for your shift, but one nurse called in sick; at the same time the recovery room has called to say that you are getting a patient, but you have no bed available. The emergency room nurse is in the middle of the nurse's station yelling for someone to listen to her report, and the ICU physician, rather belligerent, says he needs someone to assist him for a pulmonary artery line insertion (a large catheter line inserted into the venous system and through the heart to make diagnostic determination for therapeutic treatments) for the patient in bed 4. You call the nursing supervisor to obtain assistance for your unit and you are told that none is available, "you will have to make do with what you have" — four nurses for more than 10 patients. You head back to the locker room, and open your purse to reach for the aspirin for the headache which has already begun.

To most modern nurses, the preceding scenario no doubt has an uncanny ring of familiarity. For practicing professionals, this situation depicts the commonplace in almost every American hospital, in any city, in any state. Moreover, whether it be home healthcare, hospital, ambulatory care or physician office nursing, nurses are all, collectively, in a crisis situation of major proportions. For too many years now, nurses have come to know the multitudinous stresses incurred as a result of their choice of profession: long hours on their feet with no breaks; off-shift work; work on holidays and weekends; exposure to infectious disease; life and death decision-making; moral and ethical dilemmas, etc. Are these stresses simply inevitable for those who choose nursing as their career? Most nursing professionals would say, "Not so!" Instead, what is represented in the preceding scenario is **NURSE ABUSE** — the overall deterioration of a once-noble profession. The elements which comprise and which will define **NURSE ABUSE** have been in existence as long as there have been nurses. It has been recognized, both within and outside of the profession, that nurses have been and continue to be abused in a variety of ways. However, it is only with the currently tumultuous state of nursing that **NURSE ABUSE** can be recognized as a serious and disabling phenomenon, a raging cancer-like growth, threatening to consume, destroy and obliterate nursing as it now exists. In fact, **NURSE ABUSE** has ramifications so significant that it jeopardizes the healthcare profession at large, and the welfare of the general public as a whole.

Types of abuse are well-documented in the literature. The lay public knows about child abuse, woman abuse, sexual abuse, elder abuse and substance abuse. Until now, there have been only fragmented references to the "abuse" of nurses, although it is becoming more frequently recognized both inside and outside the profession. Virtually nothing has been written as a comprehensive analysis of the issue, and little has been done to correct and eradicate the problem.

It would, of course, for the sake of simplicity, be easier to contrive a one sentence definition to illustrate the term **NURSE ABUSE**; i.e. the mistreatment, neglect, exploitation and devaluation of nurses. But to do such a thing — to limit **NURSE ABUSE** to a one-line definition — would further compound the injustice itself. It is our fervent hope that this chapter will bring to the nursing and medical community, as well as the public, a greater awareness of **NURSE ABUSE** in its entirety. We will look at **NURSE ABUSE** as a disease and the forms of abuse as the symptoms. Perhaps then we will be able to reach deep within ourselves for the cure.

ONSET OF ABUSE: THE STUDENT NURSE

As is well known, women are predisposed to the position of potential and actual abuse without choice, merely as a result of their 50-50 shot at the roulette wheel of life — being born female. Luckily, however, with the great strides accomplished by the feminist movement of the preceding decades, the mistreatment, injustice and maligning of the female population, although not eliminated, has been in many instances, brought to the forefront of public awareness. As women, we are trained or conditioned to be abused, being the "weaker, subservient and emotional sex." As a result, as young ingenues entering nursing school, the seeds of abuse are already embedded and the wheels are set in motion for the onset and proliferation for what will become **NURSE ABUSE**.

Call to mind, if you can, those thoughts that blossomed during those final years in high school, that helped to make the choice of your "life's calling" to become a nurse. Your optimistic outlook and caring ideals propelled you toward the nursing role. Your goal would be one of helping people, making them better, saving lives and diminishing suffering. You envisioned yourself sitting at a dying person's bedside holding his or her hand, or comforting a crying child who awoke frightened in the middle of the night. You were well aware that needles, vomitus and bedpans constituted the non-glamorous aspects of the job, but you were prepared to meet the physical, emotional and intellectual challenges that the role of nursing would provide. Despite the fact that family members and "significant others" often questioned your career choice ("You're too smart to be a nurse, why don't you be a doctor?"), you were prepared to face the challenges you thought nursing had to offer. Little did you know when you first walked those hallowed halls of nursing academia how unprepared you were for the true job of nursing.

Regardless of their type of basic preparation (i.e., a two-three, or four-year course of study), nurses are united in their recollections of the nightmares endured in the quest to become a registered nurse (RN) or licensed practical nurse (LPN). (Unfortunately that may be *the only* element that unifies these groups.) From the students working for the institution in which she matriculates, (providing coverage for periods at any time of the day or night, any days of the week), to the pupil subjected to the "all-nighter," preparing the care plan for the next clinical day, the rigors and stressors are daunting to say the least. It is well past time to take a serious look at what we are doing to nursing students, who represent the future.

The student nurse is inaugurated into the realm of **NURSE ABUSE** the moment he or she accepts admission to an accredited school of nursing. Prior to the current crisis, when competition for entry into nursing school was fierce, only the best and brightest were fortunate enough to land a seat in the upcoming freshman class. Not only was it imperative to be academically qualified, it was also necessary to be a well-rounded and upstanding citizen, with demonstrated participation in extra-curricular activities in order to be admitted into a nursing program. These characteristics were considered essential in order to insure the greatest chance for success of the potential candidate in the program.

It is from this moment on that the novice sacrifices her individualism on the altar of the larger god—the school — adopting, for the greater part of her academic life, the school's philosophy of nursing. Categorized by her fellow university colleagues as the "poor unfortunate nursing student," she gives up her social life, corralled into classes starting at 8 a.m., and then obliged to spend endless hours after a full day of classes in the library. Usually rising at 5 a.m. to practice at the hospital, the nursing student is compelled to give up much-needed sleep in order to be prepared for clinical practice. You watch, with envy, your fellow collegians sleeping until noon after a night out on the town, or after they have attended a campus party all night. It makes you wonder whether the present sacrifices will be worth the eventual goal: that of being a nurse.

The intense academic requirements of nursing school are taken for granted by those who have endured them, but are totally unrecognized by those who have not. It is necessary to be educated in a multitude of academic disciplines — mathematics, biology, chemistry, microbiology, anatomy and physiology, pathophysiology, psychology, sociology, history, theology and philosophy, not to mention the requirements designed to make a "well-rounded student" — and all this on top of the profusion of nursing educational courses required.

Academic requirements aside, the emotional and physical stress and ethical uncertainties the nurse-ingenue is subject to are perhaps more subtle then the others and therefore less dramatic in their impact. But these are important components in the reality of nursing that are never sufficiently addressed in the academic curriculum of the nursing student. For every compassionate, empathetic nursing instructor, there is one who is just as rigid, unyielding and unsympathetic. Exposing students to the reality of the profession is one thing. But creating such a state of disequilibrium during their student years causes some to experience nervous breakdowns, eating disorders, and suicidal ideation, and that is quite another. One nursing instructor at a university emphatically spoke these words, "We will, for the next four years, put you in a constant state of disequilibrium." She was deadly serious. I'll never forget calling an all-night help line one night because a fellow nursing student had told me she was considering committing suicide after she had flunked chemistry for the third time. (This was before I had gone through my psychiatric nursing rotation when I would have learned the "correct" way to deal with this distraught person.) Does it take this type of cold, hard reality to make

us take a good, hard look at what some of us are doing to
our nursing students?

Unrealistic "testing" criteria abound in nursing
education. For example, take the student who receives a
patient assignment on Thursday evening and is expected
to prepare a full plan of care for her patient assignment
on Friday morning at 7 a.m. The result? A physically and
emotionally exhausted nursing student. One student was
told that she nearly failed her psychiatric nursing rotation,
not because of her failing a test or her poor academic performance, but "for failing to establish a therapeutic relationship" with a patient who was a chronic schizophrenic
(of 15 years duration) during her eight-week psychiatric
rotation. Another example: take the student who has
ruptured her appendix, forced to return to school within
only one week of the event because, in the school of nursing, there is no room for personal problems or misfortunes.
Miss too many clinical practices or too much classroom
work, and you will be forced out of school.

This discussion of what nursing students endure is
not meant as an attempt to criticize and censure nursing
faculty, but merely to bring to light those common practices to which the nursing student is routinely subjected
— those things that contribute to the proliferation of
NURSE ABUSE. Although it purports to illustrate the
reality of the work place, the teaching of nurses fails to
expose the student in training to the true, work-related
realities: shift rotation, weekend work, holidays, short
staffing, excessive patient-to-nurse ratios, critical care
nursing, emotional stress, ethical dilemmas and healthcare-
related business issues. With many healthcare agencies
now being run by business professionals, not healthcare
professionals, it is imperative to teach nursing students
the principles of business practice. Also, more time must
be allotted for clinical practice, even if it necessitates in-

creasing existing programs by another year.

The status of the modern nursing student in the healthcare environment is yet another subject that warrants immediate and drastic attention and intervention. It is at this formidable crossroad that nursing educators and staff personnel can jointly make or break the nursing student. The fledgling nurse needs a friendly face, a sympathetic ear, a guiding hand in those impressionable early days of practice. Too often, he or she is treated as a third-class citizen by the hospital/institutional staff, and is compelled to carry out the more unpleasant duties of the overworked and overstressed staff nurse.

Frequently, the nursing staff views the student as a hindrance rather than a help by because of the time required to explain procedures, policies and other formalities of care. "I can do it in half the time myself" — so the saying goes. Unfortunately, the student is left feeling incompetent, and in the way. Even more serious is the fact that the student is often looked at as a ready source of "an extra pair of hands," allowing administrators to lull themselves into a false sense of staffing security, and convince one another that they managed to get by without another nurse, for just another day. The profession of medicine and members of some interdisciplinary departments also prey upon the innocent nurse, who bears the brunt of their frustrations. It is sometimes made painfully evident to the student that the hospital staff does not want them there, and that patients' families do not want them there either. Another blow to the morale of the nursing student is the "You don't have it as bad as I did" attitude. The "I suffered through nursing school and so can you" sentiment, offered as if some demented "rite of passage" to the nursing profession were required, is unnecessary. By giving nursing students what they think is "reality" in the work place, some seasoned professionals are, in essence, destroying the new nurse's motivation, optimism and idealism, and undermining her emotionally, shattering her self-esteem and destroying her professional self-concept before she has ever had an opportunity to thrive and grow in her new role as a "real nurse."

PROFESSIONAL ABUSE

The trials and tribulations in the life of the student nurse prematurely place her in the fast lane of one of the most significant components of **NURSE ABUSE** itself, professional abuse. Professional abuse, for all intent and purpose, can be subdivided into three major categories: 1) Nurse-to-Nurse Abuse; 2) Physician-to-Nurse Abuse; 3) Administration-to-Nurse Abuse.

Nurse-to-Nurse Abuse

The proverbial "line of demarcation" within the nurse-to-nurse relationship begins innocently enough as the result of the nursing profession's diverse preparatory educational background: the LPN, (Licensed Practical Nurse) vs. the RN (Diploma Graduate) vs. the RN (Associate Degree) vs. the RN (Baccalaureate Degree) vs. the RN (Master's Degree). The profusion of possibilities has promoted an ongoing rift between nurses, which has been widening for years. The different programs available for educating nurses were tailored to meet the individual's personal and socio-economic needs, as well as to meet the differing caregiver needs of institutions.

In the past, the argument was made that "a nurse is a nurse is a nurse"; but present attempts to regulate entry-level educational requirements within the profession have made this mode of thinking outdated. There has always been, to some degree, dissension among nurses because of their differing educational nursing backgrounds, creating feelings of divisiveness among nurses. Frequently now, LPNs find their contribution in acute care settings increasingly valued by the institution. The RN is allegedly more cost-efficient, and JCAH (Joint Commission of Accredited Hospitals) accreditation standards require staffing which is predominantly comprised of RNs, a fact which is contributing to the demise of the role LPNs in acute care setting.

But more fundamental to this issue is the unrest among RNs. The point of view held by nursing, as a profession, seems to be that the RN with the baccalaureate or master's degree is truly the "professional" in the realm of nursing. Diploma-degree nurses argue that they are the more technically skilled, because of their superior clinical experience. The BSN nurses (baccalaureate degree) argue that, although their clinical practice may be lacking, their knowledge of theoretical principles makes them superior nurses (and they can play "catch-up" in the clinical setting). Although some may consider this supposed advantage of extensive theoretical knowledge of little practical value in day-to-day practice, it does set the stage for competition and animosity among nurses, between the BSN "haves" and the diploma "have nots." The nurse-to-nurse relationship inevitably suffers as a result, and nurse-to-nurse abuse is perpetuated from within.

What is at the root of these contentious nurse-to-nurse relationships? Is the problem intrinsic to a profession of predominately females only, the mundane business of "girls being girls"? The answer unfortunately is not that simple. Ashley (1981, p. 3) writes that nurses continue to function in a patriarchal system, one in which nursing remains contained in a sexist profession. Patriarchy has its roots clearly entrenched in misogyny, or the hatred of women; "Sexism is an obstacle to realizing full development, and perpetuates the stereotypes of femininity and masculinity. Women incorporate male values and attitudes in the patriarchal system, and devalue other women's performances, attitudes, goals, and backgrounds" (Reakes, 1981, p. 8). Therein lies the dilemma.

With its origin in patriarchy, nursing has continued to imitate and then perpetuate male behaviors and attitudes. Thus, nurse-to-nurse abuse continues to thrive. As a result, we are unable to realize our full potential, that of governing and controlling our profession, being at the helm of what transpires within the profession. Functioning in the sphere of a male-dominated profession — medicine — nurses do continue to serve physicians and administrators. Their feelings of frustration and powerlessness in this role cause them to ventilate their frustration and rage on that easily accessible target, the other nurse. But is it necessary to consider this behavior as being inseparable from the profession?

As previously mentioned, the seeds of nurse-to-nurse abuse are planted within the student nurses, as they are introduced into the profession. Another example is what happens to the "new" staff nurse. Territorialism may be instinctive behavior, but with the addition of the new staff member to the nursing unit, the existing staff sometimes goes out of its way to make her feel, quite bluntly, miserable. The new nurse is usually evaluated against some hidden testing criteria in order to prove herself worthy to join the ranks.

First impressions are of the utmost importance in helping people decide whether or not they will stay in a particular position. This type of initiation is obviously not a way to establish positive first impressions. A different and more understanding approach could help considerably in decreasing one major component of the current crisis — staff turnover.

Scapegoating is another commonly employed strategy in the nurse-to-nurse abuse syndrome. Let's face it. We are all, at one time or another, guilty of gossiping, placing blame elsewhere, or taking our frustrations out on other staff members. Because of the serious constraints imposed upon nurses by the present nursing shortage, we frequently find ourselves falling short of our own personal and professional expectations with respect to the kind of care we want to deliver to our patients. As a result, we place blame elsewhere — on each other. Our colleagues bear the brunt of our frustrations. How many times have we rolled our eyes in disgust when we found out we were taking report from Nurse Whomever, the one who always leaves her rooms like disaster areas, with her patients in a pre-code condition having "things-to-do" lists a mile long? Immediately addressing such interpersonal professional practice problems with those involved may help to defuse the intra-departmental conflicts which so often ignite at these stressful times — times in which inadequate staffing, insufficient and aging equipment, more critically ill patients and lack of administrative support are commonplace.

The "generally competent" nurse (one who is able to function in a general medical-surgical setting, but unable to function adequately in a particular specialty area) is not commonly addressed in the nursing administrative arena. The "generally competent" nurse is that nurse who does not or cannot practice in a prudent, knowledgeable and professional manner as compared to that of her peers in a specialty setting. This, after every educational and training opportunity has been afforded to that nurse. An example of this is the nurse who makes a terrific medical-surgical nurse, but is unable to switch areas of expertise and become an equally skilled intensive care unit nurse. In light of past, present and probable future nursing shortages, this issue has been and may continue to be a major source of persistent nurse-to-nurse abuse. Because of chronic shortages in specialty areas, administrators have preferred to turn a deaf ear to stated concerns that a given nurse may not be equipped to handle responsibilities in a particular specialty area. It's far easier to think in terms of that "warm body" that has, finally, filled that chronically vacant staffing slot. Not enough attention is given to this occurrence. The already overstressed and competent nurse situation is physically, emotionally and intellectually unable to compensate for the shortcomings of the generally competent nurse who cannot keep pace with her peers in the specialty unit. It's unfair to all concerned, and it's one more — albeit subtle — example of nurse-to-nurse abuse.

Physician-to-Nurse Abuse

The nurse/physician relationship is frequently discussed, frequently dissected and frequently lamented. Throughout the history of medicine, there has been a symbiotic relationship between nurses and physicians in which medicine has ultimately dominated. Although emancipated, to a certain degree, from the "handmaiden mentality," "the control, domination, intimidation and nullification of individual will implicit in a system of medical patriarchy generates many nurses who do not recognize their abusive situation" (Lovell, 1981 p. 25).

Every day, in some way, shape or form, nurses continue to be abused by physicians. In a survey of nurse-physician relationships by Friedman (1982, p. 39), it was concluded that nurses face a multitude of abuses from their non-nurse healthcare colleagues:

1) condescending attitudes
2) lack of respect as either a person or professional
3) public humiliation, as physicians rant and rave in front of patients, families or anyone who will listen

    4) temper tantrums (MDs who scream and throw things if unhappy about anything)

    5) scapegoating — nurses are often blamed for anything that goes wrong, or are easy targets if the doctor is merely "in a bad mood"

    6) failure to read nurses' notes or listen to nurses' suggestions

    7) refusal to share information about the patient

    8) lack of understanding about what nurses do

    9) frequent disparaging remarks in public (Cox, 1987, p. 47).

Imagine what would happen if a nurse were guilty of the same abuse behavior. It would never be tolerated! So why, then, do physicians continue demonstrating these behaviors without reproach? Nurses themselves must bear part of the responsibility for the perpetuation of nurse abuse by physicians. Although having evolved from the "servant" role to the "interdisciplinary team member," nurses continue to maintain their significance in patient care delivery at a level lower than that of the all-knowing, all-healing physician. Nurses are co-professionals to physicians, their primary responsibility being *to the patient.* The nurse's role is that of patient advocate, and she directs her responsibility and care to the patient, not to the physician. Her primary purpose is to be accountable for all facets of the patient's care — not be at the beck and call of the physician.

Administrative Abuse of Nurses

As significant as the abuse of nurses is by physicians and other nurses, the phenomenon of **NURSE ABUSE** by administrator/administration is virtually unequalled. Once the intrinsic grievances of the profession have been verbalized — those of wages, hours, staffing and respect — the cornerstone to **NURSE ABUSE** (and that which bears the brunt of the responsibility), is the healthcare institution. Those who represent the bureaucratic, business-suit mentality, comfortably seated in the upholstered chair behind the slick mahogany desk, are primarily responsible for the static state of the nursing profession today.

The administrative abuse of nurses emerges as the single most important, widespread and commonly identified element found in surveys of nursing job satisfaction. Nurses, who are equipped to make, and should be empowered to make, decisions regarding optimal, holistic patient care, are fiscally being held hostage by their institutions. Their ability to implement change, to deliver the type of nursing care of which they are capable (and which their patients deserve), are all limited by budgetary constraints.

With the advent in recent years of DRGs (Diagnostic Related Groupings), the assault on the nursing profession has become even more intense. Nursing positions have been cut, and lay-offs or defections have occurred at the very same time that hospital administrators are rewarded with company cars for their due diligence in "balancing the budget." Nursing has become the "easy" solution for administrative hatchet men and women. When things get tough, nursing is inevitably singled out for staffing cutbacks. Amazingly enough, there seems to be a continued increase in the numbers and salaries of administrative positions, inspiring the often-quoted platitude, heard frequently among nurses: "There are too many chiefs and not enough Indians."

What the business-mogul administrators did not count on, however, was that DRGs would lead to both a sicker and older patient population. Increased technology has enabled the healthcare system to save more patients, coming as a direct result of increased technical skill, and ever more sophisticated diagnostic and therapeutic treatment modalities, significantly enhancing patient longevity.

Many hospitals, rather than realizing a greater profit by increasing their patient turnover, have found that DRGs have ironically led them to an increased need for skilled nurses specialized in the care of those sicker patients who are confined to institutions for longer periods of time.

The distorted administrator mentality is fiercely committed to pursuit of the almighty dollar. New hospital wings, improved diagnostic facilities and advancement in healthcare services all help the institution toward the attainment of financial viability and governmental grants. The institution's public image, achieved through aggressive community advertisement and promotion, is believed to be of the utmost importance in its ability to achieve economic superiority. It is no wonder, then, that competition between healthcare facilities is so fierce, and that they are all striving to attract the healthcare consumer.

Who will be first in line to suffer at the hands of these bureaucratic tyrants? The patients will. Who, then, is destined to follow next in line? The nurses, in their positions as the largest employed component of the healthcare industry. And so, before the present nursing crisis has even peaked, the healthcare industry finds itself in quite a quandary. Currently, there are insufficient numbers of nurses, and the demand is expected to rise over the next 10 years, leading the public into a twenty-first century in which the health-care industry will be inundated with even more elderly patients, and an unprecedented number of people afflicted with AIDS (acquired immunodeficiency syndrome) in epidemic proportions.

The financial constraints imposed upon nurses by their employers have been thoroughly documented. Wages and benefits are major contributing factors to **NURSE ABUSE**, money being the figurative guillotine held over nurses' heads by administration. Hospitals have failed to be creative in using benefit-packaging structures to reduce the escalating nursing turnover rate, and which could also lead to increased employee loyalty.

Administrators of both healthcare in general and nursing in particular recognize the legitimate power within the nursing profession. By patronizing nurses as if they were whining children, and by perpetuating the subservient, handmaiden mentality, administrators have been able to rob nurses of their legitimate power; i.e., both their numbers and their talents. To attain the position of significance that they so justly deserve in the healthcare setting, nurses must unite, whether in structured, unionized groups, or as members of those organizations in the nursing profession which are addressing important issues with seriousness and clout. Administrative managers, and nursing administration itself keep nurses bickering and fighting amongst themselves in order to keep the masses off balance and ineffectual — the classic "divide and conquer" mentality. Their total lack of respect for the nursing profession is obvious in the ways in which they refuse to allow input by nurses in nursing-related issues. In addition, rather than spending money to keep the institution's nurses content and optimally functional by improving wages, ancillary services and benefit "perks," administrators will spend millions of dollars to prevent nurses from unionizing. Clearly, they recognize the potential power in unionization, and fear a serious lack of control over nurses who are unionized.

The continued and abhorrent misuse of the nurse in the hospital setting is amply illustrated by the variety of roles the nurse is expected to assume everyday. It is taken for granted, from an administrative standpoint, that these additional roles will be carried out and performed by the nursing staff, roles that lie *outside* the realm of what nursing truly is. For instance:

1) *The nurse as the housekeeper:* The nurse is frequently responsible for moving and cleaning furniture, beds especially, in order to accept more patients, thereby increasing hospital revenue. Overflowing waste baskets are nursing's responsibility. Dusting and cleaning patient care areas, cleaning monitors and equipment — all fall under the realm of nursing duties, by default.

2) *The nurse as the secretary/clerical worker:* Nurses must answer the phone, order supplies and call different departments to track down those supplies which are much needed by the patient. Filling out lab slips, tracking down lab reports, filing lab reports and making out diagnostic procedure forms (and then obtaining results) are also mandatory for the nurse. Contacting other departments to get things accomplished is another task which is taken for granted. Voluminous paperwork, resulting from commonly found lack of computerization in the healthcare industry, contributes greatly to the clerical role imposed upon nursing.

3) *The nurse as the transporter/moving company:* Nurses spend valuable time and energy moving patients to and from wheelchairs, stretchers and beds, transporting patients to other departments, to other floors, and out the door. The time spent looking for those vehicles on/in which to transport patients is another misuse of personnel. Furniture moving has already been mentioned.

4) *The nurse as the dietitian, physical therapist, respiratory therapist, lab technician:* The nurse ensures that the appropriate diet is ordered for the appropriate patient three times a day. Because of insufficient staffing in other patient care areas, nurses have frequently been compelled to perform the duties of the physical and respiratory therapist, as well as the venipuncturist, dietitian, social worker, etc.

5) *The nurse as the police officer/security guard:*

Nurses are required to monitor the number of visitors, the frequency of visitors and the length of time the visitors stay with patients.

6) *The nurse as the handywoman:* Nurses, of necessity, have become quite versatile in their ability to troubleshoot and fix malfunctioning equipment; they've become equally adept at teaching the engineering and maintenance departments how to troubleshoot and fix malfunctioning equipment.

7) *The nurse as the nursing supervisor:* Everyday, nurses evaluate patient care needs, deciding how many staff nurses are needed to care for how many patients. The irony here is that they must then substantiate and explain their decisions to the *real* nursing supervisor. So far removed from patient care is the "nurse administrator," she should be forever indebted to the nurses at the front line who help perform her job adequately. It is the bedside nurse who is, in reality, the *true* nursing supervisor.

NURSE ABUSE is further fostered by nursing executives and managers (nursing administrators collectively), who dictate nursing practice. By utilizing computer software which cranks out data entitled "patient acuity" — a numerical value given to designate the amount of care patients require — nursing executives and managers sit behind their desks and decide how many nurses there should be to take care of "x" numbers of patients. However, this data measures routine tasks nurses perform, and does not account for the unexpected situations (e.g., emergencies, family interactions, preparation for transportation of patients for diagnostic procedures, etc.) which occur frequently in nursing. It is obvious that decisions about patient care should be made by those at the bedside, the staff nurses, not nursing administrators, who by merely reading a patient's name and diagnosis from a report sheet feel they are entitled to dictate the level of nursing care delivered to the patients on the floor. The nursing supervisory team is dependent upon the patient acuity system, taking the information as being true without even assessing the real situation, and evaluating the amount of care actually required by patients. This is, to say the least, demeaning, and only continues to contribute to the flagrant demoralization of the nursing profession.

Another problem area relative to nursing administration is the administrators' faulty perception of the realities of nursing practice — their belief is that nurses are interchangeable, that an emergency room nurse can just as easily work on a pediatric unit "in a pinch." Although it is the administrator's job to ensure the delivery of safe patient care, and although safe patient care *is* usually delivered, it is frequently at the nurse's expense. Thus, more often than not, the solution to less-than-safely-staffed patient care areas is the game we fondly refer to as "Float-the-Nurse."

Specifically, "Float the Nurse" game is played when a nurse who normally works on one unit, or in one patient care area, gets sent to another area to provide for adequate nursing coverage. If she is "lucky", that nurse will be sent to an area similar to that in which she practices. Many times, however, this is not the case. This situation can and does have serious legal ramifications. Although nurses have a basic education foundation in common, nursing has become far more diversified and specialized. As a result, the nurse can jeopardize both her career and license by working in an area in which she lacks appropriate training. For example, consider the medical-surgical nurse who gets sent to the intensive care unit to cover staffing requirements, or the intensive care unit nurse who gets sent to the nursery to work. In addition, the nurse who gets "floated" is usually the one with a higher level of nursing skill and expertise. The higher the level of expertise, the more frequently that nurse is abused by the institution to fill in the empty "slots" where nurses are needed for understaffed areas. Increased levels of knowledge in nursing practice do not necessarily make it safer for the patient if the nurse caring for him is practicing in an area not within the realm of her experience. This seems to matter little to nursing supervisory personnel.

Yet another dangerous and negligent practice among the administrative hierarchy is the popular game called the "Revolving Door." In many institutions, little concern is given to the numbers of patients, the type of nursing care required and the number of nurses needed to deliver such care. Instead, the object of the game is *fill the beds.* It is, after all, bad business practice to turn patients away, even if the bed are full to capacity. By filling the hallways, doubling patients up in what is supposed to be single-patient rooms, or sending patients out of the intensive care unit in the middle of the night, the hospital can increase patient census, and consequently increase revenue. Again, the nurse is the last to be considered. Hospital and nursing administrator insist that "it doesn't look good to the public" to close emergency rooms to patient admissions, or to transfer patients to another healthcare facility that is able to accommodate an extra patient. No concern whatsoever is given to the number of nurses available to insure safe patient care in these environments. "We don't have enough nurses!", the charge nurse will state emphatically to the nursing supervisor. The supervisor, in turn, will usually respond with a perfunctory, "You'll have to make do with what you have — you should be able to handle that many patients." In this situation, psychological warfare explodes. Nurses are made to feel that, if they are "good nurses," they should be able to care for their assigned patients, no matter how many there are.

On the other hand, some hospital or nursing administrators are telling practicing professionals that their levels of nursing practice are too high. There is no greater slap in the face than to be told by the director of nursing that "you girls need to re-evaluate your standards of practice. They are too high. Nursing is changing!"

What is the price, then, of human life? If it were the loved one of the hospital or nursing administrator lying in that hospital bed, there would not be any standard of care too high for them. Are nurses, then, destined to lower their level of practice, spreading themselves ever thinner among ever larger numbers of patients in order to ensure that the institution's tallies at the end of the fiscal year are "in the black"? It is about time that levels of nursing care be determined *by nurses!* Enough is enough — no longer should these financial henchmen and women be permitted to perpetuate these heinous and abusive acts against nurses and patients.

PHYSICAL AND ENVIRONMENTAL ABUSE OF NURSES

Nurses physically abused? Preposterous ... or is it? Certainly, there may not be broken bones, unsightly scars, blackened eyes or any of the other physical signs often seen in someone who is the victim of physical abuse or violence. The physical abuse of nurses is so much more subtle and insidious. Unfortunately, not enough attention is focused on yet another form of **NURSE ABUSE**.

Far too many nurses have known the reality of the most frequently identified hazard in the job of professional nursing — back injury. Long hours on their feet and extended overtime shifts contribute significantly to the wear and tear on the bodies of nurses. Coupled with insufficient numbers of staff available for assistance, and the lack of equipment to mobilize patients, it is inevitable that back injuries occur. One study estimated that in the span of one hour's work, two nurses lifted the equivalent of two and one half *tons* of patient weight on the nursing unit on which they worked. In another study "of more than 500 staff nurses, 52% said they had work-related back pain that lasted longer than 14 days. These nurses were young. (83% were under the age of 30.) Those who had suffered from back pain traced it to three activities: lifting a patient in bed, helping a patient get out of bed, and moving a bed" (Gates, 1988, p. 656). Moreover, wherever there is a shortage of nurses, injuries flourish, all despite the conscientious use of proper body mechanics.

Although back injury is the most common injury to nurses, other orthopedic problems are well documented. Injuries such as cervical strain, tendinitis, foot and leg ailments, varicosities and corns occur frequently. And what becomes of these ill-fated nurses who have the audacity to become injured? They are labeled by the institution or agency for which they work as liabilities. From the institutional perspective of risk management, the injured nurse is just that — a *risk*. Rather than investigate the causative event and variables, the institution interprets the injury as being the fault of the nurse, and any responsibility for the physical damage should be sustained by the worker. Furthermore, when it comes to the issue of monetary compensation for illness or injury incurred on the job, nurses get a raw deal because they are seen as being dispensable. It would behoove healthcare institutions to spend money on such necessities as patient-lifting equipment and ancillary staff to help move patients, or safely staff nursing units with *more* nurses. From a risk management perspective, these remedies, in and of themselves, would help to decrease the numbers of work-related injuries and hence, decrease the number of expenditures related to Workmen's Compensation.

Another seldom-discussed but prevalent form of physical abuse sustained by nurses is the result of the combative patient. Ask any emergency room nurse on a Saturday night shift if she is physically abused. You will hear a resounding *yes!* Ask any psychiatric nurse, ask any medical-surgical nurse — the list goes on and on. Physical injury to nurses occurs at the hands of the confused, the bereaved, the psychotic or the drug or alcohol-intoxicated patient. Abuse consists of harm to the nurse in the form of punches, kicks, strangulation attempts, human bites and scratches. The literature discusses ways in which to handle physically abusive and potentially life-threatening patients, but there is not enough discussion with regard to the types of abuse and its statistical frequency.

Some time ago, I was engaged in conversation at a social event, discussing the subject of **NURSE ABUSE**. The man with whom I was speaking encouraged me to expand upon the ways in which nurses are abused. When I cited physical abuse, he stopped me in my tracks, "Physical abuse? Nurses are physically abused?" he asked incredulously. When I began describing the combative patient, he stopped me from continuing once again. "Well, isn't that a part of your job?" he asked. "Combative patients are a work-related hazard, a part of what your pay compensates you for," he told me. "You get paid to take it!" After a 30 minute discussion he relinquished his hold on his ill-conceived idea, indebted for his newly found insights. Unfortunately, he was and is not alone in his ignorance. It is a philosophy shared by far too many. Nurses need to make people aware.

Shift work, a mandatory component of the nursing profession, is also a contributory factor to the physical abuse of nursing. Much has been written about circadian rhythms, and the effect that shift rotation plays on the body's intrinsic biological time clock. "Studies have shown that after several years of rotating shifts, worker's general health problems appear earlier than in [those who are] straight day workers. Other studies have proved that gastrointestinal disease occurs earlier in three-shift workers, and that the incidence of myocardial infarction relates directly to the amount of exposure to shift work" (Janowski, 1988, p. 1337). People require nursing care 24 hours a day, seven days a week, 52 weeks a year, so it is impossible for shift work to become obsolete. It would, though, make shift work less physically detrimental if employers would follow guidelines and recommendations proposed by researchers and experts in the fields related to sleep and circadian rhythms. "Based on a review of research into various shift-rotation systems, sleep expert Torbjorn Akerstedt of Sweden suggests several shift strategies; a short night shift (six to eight hours), clockwise rotation (days to evenings to nights) with nights at the end of the series, and a slow rotation (four to seven days)" (Janowski, 1988, p. 1341).

As a rather unfortunate reflection of the times, mandatory overtime is becoming a more frequent means of staffing understaffed units. Many times a nurse is required to work a double shift if staffing is inadequate. Not only is mandatory overtime sanctioned in contractual language, the guilt-induced obligatory contract within the mind of the nurse causes her to be unable to turn her back and abandon the short-staffed nursing unit on which patient lives may be in jeopardy. It is not only physically exhausting to work 16 consecutive hours in a high-pressured job, it may also prove dangerous. In a situation where the nurse needs her judgment to be flawless, her physical condition also plays a major role. A nurse (or any person for that matter,) is more apt to make an error, or to overlook a crucial observation if she is physically exhausted. In a profession where an error can cause serious or fatal consequences, working under these conditions jeopardizes not only the nurse's license, but even more importantly the patient's very welfare. And what of "break" times mandated by law for working eight hours on the job? These necessary rest periods are becoming fewer and farther between, as nurses find it nearly impossible to take the much needed break time, because there simply are no people available to relieve them. Rather than pay staff members who are compelled to work through their allotted break time, more and more facilities have chosen to eliminate the "break" by shortening off-shifts to eight hours only. The nursing staff is, therefore, entitled to only a five-to-10 minute break every four hours, as determined by their state laws. In addition, the eight-hour shift inevitably becomes nine, 10 hour shifts become 11 in length, and 12 hour shifts extend to 13, as nurses stay late, often without remuneration, striving to accomplish everything required by their patients, but unable to finish during their allotted shifts. Budgetary compliance being a must, institutions require nurses to all but prostitute themselves, figuratively speaking, to receive compensation for total hours worked. This is illustrated in the example of the institution which requires the nurse to notify her supervisor that she will not be finished on time, to fill out a form stating the reason for the "tardiness", and to have it approved by the nursing supervisor. If this protocol is not followed, the nurse does not receive payment for the overtime worked. For the nurse who doesn't finish her work on time, a slap on the wrist is in order and she is told by the supervisory personnel that she is incapable of utilizing her time efficiently.

One final bone of contention among nurses with regard to shift work is the ever-elusive goal of permanent steady day shift hours once the status of seniority has been achieved. Nurses continue to be scheduled to work both the day and night shifts in a five day work week and, hence, the perpetuation of the physical abuse of nurses continues.

These are the overt physical dangers to nurses in the hospital environment. But what of the less obvious ones — those that lurk in every nook and cranny of the hospital and healthcare facility? According to one estimate (Leonard, 1988, p. 59), "60 percent" of all healthcare workers are regularly exposed to numerous toxic chemicals, ranging from the obvious dangers— such as formaldehyde, used in the lab and morgue, to common cleaning solutions, used all over the hospital everyday." And what of the other hazards: x-ray machines, radiation implants, testing with radioisotopes or anesthetic gases which nurses come in contact with, whether knowingly or not? All pose serious health risks to workers. X-ray machines can cause genetic malformations, sterility or cancer. Exposure to certain drugs can cause those who handle them adverse effects, cytotoxic and chemotherapeutic agents the most devastating offenders. Something as seemingly benign as bone cement, used in the operating room during orthopedic procedures, can cause respiratory tract ailments, and can be potentially carcinogenic.

Bacterial and viral agents are abundant in the healthcare environment. Exposure through blood, sputum and excrement results in nurses being vulnerable to infectious or contagious diseases. The increased occurrence of hepatitis B is well documented. However, many institutions continue to refuse to vaccinate their employees against this debilitating disease. The AIDS epidemic has had a profound impact on nursing. Healthcare workers take a risk, not so much with the diagnosed patient but with the undiagnosed. A major shift in behavior and thinking is necessary in order to consider everyone as being potentially infectious.

In 1985 (Bennett, 1985, p. 968), a surveillance of 722 healthcare workers with documented exposure to blood or body fluids of patients with AIDS revealed the majority of exposed workers were nurses; doctors and lab workers also report exposure. Seventy-nine percent of exposures were in patient care areas. The most frequent (85%) exposures are to blood, (74% parenterally, 15% to mucous membranes, and 11% to open wounds); then saliva and respiratory secretions. "The CDC (Center for Disease Control) projects that the risk to healthcare workers is small. They also claim that isolation recommendations are adequate" regarding safe handling and disposal of sharp instruments, thereby preventing unnecessary exposure (Bennett, 1988, p. 971). But how safe do you feel coming in contact with these infectious body fluids? How many individuals do you know take such a risk in caring for a total stranger?

Fortunately, OSHA (Occupational Safety and Health Administration) has expanded regulations to cover hospital workers on the job. The "right-to-know" regulations compel hospitals to enact programs for employees to be informed of the work environment hazards they are exposed to (Leonard, 1988, p. 59). "Among these rights given to hospital employees by the OSHA regulations are these:

• The right to have a material safety data sheet — it describes the contents of a product and the hazards involved in its use — provided on request.

• The right to receive thorough education about potentially hazardous chemicals you may come in contact with.

• The right to have appropriate personnel protective equipment — goggles, face masks or respirators, for example — available for you to use when handling these chemicals" (Leonard, 1988, p. 59).

Healthcare workers must know their rights and

make their institution responsible for providing this information to them.

Physically and environmentally speaking, the poor design and structure of nursing units or patient care areas is another example of **NURSE ABUSE**. Billions of dollars are spent for the architectural designs and construction of "state-of-the-art" healthcare facilities. But, again, without significant input from those very people who work in those areas most frequently ... *nurses!* Cramming the greatest number of people into the smallest possible space for the least amount of money seems to be the institution's goal. As an example, a six bed surgical intensive care unit was converted to an 11 bed mixed medical-surgical intensive care unit in an institution in which I was employed. Sounds like an impossible task, doesn't it? It was accomplished, however. Serious attempts should be made to take into account the environmental as well as physical needs of the nurses who are to staff those units. With nurses working 24 hours a day in these areas, their opinions and recommendations with regard to design and construction should be given the highest possible consideration.

EMOTIONAL AND ETHICAL STRESSES AND ABUSE

Few other professionals experience the breadth of human emotions felt by the registered professional nurse. Few, too, are confronted by the ethical decision-making dilemmas which are regularly thrust upon nurses each day. The emotional stress and ethical agonizing which nurses must face day in and day out are substantial contributors to **NURSE ABUSE** in general. Nurses make difficult and sophisticated decisions regarding the patients they care for based on sound scientific, psychological, emotional and ethical principles. Being confronted regularly with such momentous responsibilities (frequently of life and death import), there exists the potential for serious psychological abuse of nurses. There is, at best, an extremely fine line between what some will describe and interpret as stress, and what others will describe and interpret as abuse. It is therefore necessary to make a clear distinction between that which constitutes each as they relate to nursing.

The emotional components of patient care, and of the interactions with the patient's family contribute to the emotional stress of the nurse simply because he or she is "involved." Nurses have the same emotions as any other human beings, and they inevitably become attached to their patients and/or families. As a result, when the patient suffers from an irreversible disease, the nurse, too, can suffer. The nurse "hurts," the nurse cries, the nurse mourns — just as any other sensitive person would under these traumatic circumstances. Although nurses are usually portrayed as hard, emotionless or cold human beings, they experience the same feelings as anyone else. As an example, patients feed on the nurse's emotions in an insidious and subtle way, by making her feel responsible for their psychological and emotional needs, as well as for the outcome of their physical well being (and, by extension, for their discomfort and pain, bad hospital food, lack of supplies, lack of progress). Families of the patient, in another way, also contribute to the emotional burden suffered by nurses. "Save my loved one, help me decide what to do, help me with the doctor," they will ask. There is no doubt that it is difficult to deal with disease, suffering and death on a daily basis. Nursing encompasses so many different facets: helping to bring a child into the world, saving a life, easing the pain of the dying. It is little wonder that nurses are emotionally drained and stressed. It comes with the territory. We know that when we become nurses we will have to deal with and shoulder a variety of emotional experiences inherent in caring for people. By citing the emotional stress placed on nurses by patients and their families, I am not attempting to place blame; rather, I am simply pointing out some of the contributing factors to the emotional stressors confronting the nurse.

In light of the present state of nursing, another type of emotional stress is evident. The nursing shortage has forced nurses to cut corners in order to save time, taking care of larger numbers of sicker patients. As a result, nurses experience feelings of inadequacy from trying to fulfill all the needs of their patients, and being unable to accomplish this. Nurses feel anger and rage at those who attempt to undermine their goals and their idealism. In this type of environment, nurses vent their frustrations on other nurses, blaming each other for their respective inadequacies. Backstabbing and scapegoating then become instinctive behaviors, leading to even more heightened levels of emotional stress for the nurses to cope with. This stress is further fueled by nursing supervisory personnel (or administrators) who, rather than provide support to the stressed nurses, compound the problems by making light of the emotions the nurses feel in these types of situations ... "So, you can't take care of the patient the way you want to — you have to be realistic," or, "Nurse Jones seems a little burned out lately, do you think she needs to change jobs?" or, "If you were an efficient nurse, you'd be able to finish your work on time."

With regard to the actual emotional abuse of nurses, there are primarily two major culprits: nursing administrators and physicians. With regard to nursing administration, take, for example, the nurse who is ill and calls in sick — not a cut-and-dried matter, as it would appear to be, since the nurse is sure to receive a guilt-inducing description of the status of the unit she is leaving inadequately staffed, unable to "serve." "Oh, no, there will only be two nurses for 50 patients," the supervisor will say. "You're leaving us short staffed, I won't be able to find anyone to replace you. Are you sure you can't come to work?" The same kind of emotional abuse is experienced by the nurse attempting to take time off for a vacation, or by the nurse who refuses to do an overtime shift. Inevitably, the most blatant emotional abuse and manipulation ensues. The nurse is made to feel irresponsible and guilty. She is made to suffer because she has deprived her fellow nurses and her patients by her "selfishness."

Physicians contribute to nurses' emotional stress and abuse in a number of ways and, more frequently than not, it is abuse that typifies the physician-nurse relationship from physicians to nurses (in addition to the emotional stress that is sustained). Physicians scream at nurses (a form of verbal as well as emotional abuse); insult them ("Find me someone around here that knows what they're doing"); belittle them in front of colleagues and others ("I'm the doctor!"); and patronize them. One physician said to a colleague of mine, "You girls need to learn the difference between medicine and nursing; when was the last time you gave a backrub?" If they don't take the nurse's concerns about the patient seriously, they ignore the nurse, offending both her intelligence and expertise. They accuse nurses of being "too emotional," and of not being able to be objective about the patient, interpreting the nurse's genuine empathy and emotion as "unprofessional" (while exhibiting little if any emotion themselves). These types of behaviors by physicians feed into the already diminished sense of worth nurses have, and tend to make them think they are, indeed, less worthy, less contributory, etc.; their opinions, philosophies, feelings and perceptions less valid than those of the "more important" healthcare worker ... the doctor himself.

With the technological advances and diagnostic sophistication in the field of medicine, the population grows older and lives longer. As a result, nurses are faced with ever more frequent, ethically charged and emotionally wrought dilemmas, providing the perfect medium for what can be considered "ethical stress." In her everyday practice, the nurse plays a virtual tug-of-war with herself, trying to make the "right" decision for her patients. For example, consider the patient who begs his nurse to allow him to die. Frequently, the family or physician (or both) refuse to "give up" on the patient so to speak, and allow nature to take its course. The nurse is bound to uphold the wishes of the family and the physician, or be faced with possible legal consequences. The patient's wishes are often ignored, and the nurse is compelled to "save" the patient by instituting resuscitative or invasive procedures. This, despite the fact that the patient may have communicated otherwise. It must be remembered that nurses spend 24 hours a day caring for the patient and they witness the suffering on a far more consistent basis, and they see patients at their worst, whereas doctors and families spend only a relatively small portion of time with the patient, usually after the patient is made to look "comfortable" and "presentable" as possible. This is just one more example of the emotional stress nurses sustain.

The responsibility nurses feel for policing other members of the healthcare team, particularly physicians, is another example of an ethics-associated stressor. The nurse must ensure that all physician's orders are appropriate, that procedures are carried out with the utmost of care and technical skill, and that any incompetencies are reported. Once, in an intensive care unit in which I worked, a staff nurse brought to the attention of a staff physician that a physician still in training had performed a minor invasive procedure with less-than-optimal sterile procedure. The nurse believed this to be a matter of some significance to this patient who was already very ill, and highly susceptible to infection. The doctor's response to the nurse: "Well if you *girls* hadn't asked the resident to perform the procedure there wouldn't have been any problem! It's your fault!" It would appear that by doing what is right, the nurse is often found to be wrong. The fine line that exists between ethical stress and abuse is crossed when, after questioning a physician's order that the nurse knows from her knowledge and experience to be incorrect, she is told by the physician to carry it out regardless. She has two options in this situation: to either carry out the order or procedure which she knows to be wrong, or refuse to do so and be ready to face the consequences of her "insubordination." This situation illustrates ethical abuse.

An additional thought-provoking example of the ethical abuse of nurses is the following: You are the charge nurse on a nursing unit. You are already dangerously understaffed for the number of patients you have, and the complexity of care that they require. You are called by the emergency room and told you will be receiving two more very sick patients. You know you can't possibly accept two more patients without receiving more nursing personnel. You notify your nursing supervisor/administrator who tells you there are no additional nurses available for assistance. You tell her you can't possibly accept these patients. She tells you that you have no choice, you must admit these patients to your floor, there are no empty beds in the hospital. The dynamics of this situation lead to ethical abuse for several different reasons. The nurse is being abused as a result of being forced to do what she knows is wrong. She is potentially putting her nursing license as well as her personal integrity and principles on the line, not to mention the lives of the patients she and the other nurses she works with are caring for. That's wrong. The right thing to do would be to admit these patients because they need and deserve medical care. The wrong thing to do is to give less-than-sufficient nursing care, as well as jeopardize lives. It would also be ethically wrong for her to threaten to leave, thereby threatening to "abandon" her patients. This all-too-common occurrence illustrates a dilemma in which the nurse involved is being ethically (as well as emotionally and professionally) abused.

Discussion of the emotional and ethical stressors and abuse nurses evidence is certainly controversial. While emotional stress and abuse may occur independently to that of ethical stress and abuse, the ethical components are inextricably intertwined with emotional elements. Two rather simple strategies to address these issues might be inclusions of courses of ethics study in nursing curricula, and having functioning ethics committees in healthcare settings where nurses practice. With respect to the emotional component of abuse, the continued intentional humiliation of nurses must cease. If not, the practicing nursing population will continue to dwindle, as more and more nurses become the victims of burnout from **NURSE ABUSE** — and as fewer and fewer of them remain willing to put up with it.

THE FINANCIAL ABUSE OF NURSES

The following provides a brief overview of the types of financial abuses nurses endure. The solutions to these abuses are evident. Only active, informed and involved nurses can effect change with regard to the injustices of this component of **NURSE ABUSE.**

1) *Wages and Raises*

Despite salary gains, especially in the past few years, there is still a definite lack of adequate compensation for the number of years of experience and longevity of professional nurses in the healthcare system. Comparatively, nursing has failed to keep step with other professions in salary growth. Additionally, nurses are often at the mercy of their employers with regard to raises. If no bargaining unit contract is in existence, nursing salaries are governed by merit raises or cost of living increases at best; at one hospital without a contract, nurses had no raise in an 18 month period. Many readers may know of even more outrageous financial abuses.

2) *Benefits and "Perks"*

In this area, the old adage, "You don't get something for nothing" holds true — a virtual trade-off ensues. In order to enjoy increased hourly or weekly wages, nurses often find their benefit packages progressively chipped away in order to find such increases. Decreases in such benefits as tuition reimbursement and holiday pay often follow. Finally, decreases in employer payment of health insurance premiums may be the final sacrifice nurses must make in order to obtain increased wages.

3) *Educational Reimbursements*

It has been well-documented that the educational loan program through the federal government has suffered a substantial decline over the past several years. It is only with the current nursing shortage that some nursing education support programs and loans have been reenacted by legislators. Institutional tuition reimbursement has frequently fallen by the wayside. Advanced nursing degrees and certification in nursing specialty areas are also not monetarily compensated in many areas of healthcare, despite professional and administrative pressure to achieve higher levels of educational and professional expertise. In addition, in order to obtain nursing licensure renewal, it is mandated that nurses show proof of continuing education units (CEUs) and seminar attendance. Often, payment for these programs comes right out of the nurse's own pocket. If any reimbursement to nurses is given at all, it is dependent upon the good graces of the institution or healthcare agency.

4) *Child Care*

Unfortunately, the employers of nurses still fall considerably behind other businesses in providing on-site child care services for their employees. Shift work, notoriously associated with the nursing profession, makes it extremely difficult to find suitable child care services within the community. The continued inflexibility of work schedules and lack of creative staffing patterns in healthcare agencies also contributes significantly to the financial abuse of nurses with regard to the obtaining of child care services.

5) *Agency or Temporary Nurses*

Healthcare facilities continue to pay exorbitant fees for agency nurses, those versatile individuals who are able to "plug in" to any institution at any particular time to meet staffing demands. It remains a bone of contention for the hospital staff nurse to work side by side with an agency nurse who, many times, is earning double the hourly wage. If institutions would pay their own nursing staff more money and increase ancillary services, they would improve job satisfaction among their own employees and thereby increase employee loyalty.

6) *The Clinical Ladder or Career Ladder*

This is one of the more recent attempts to "keep nurses happy." Additional dollars in the form of a percentage of hourly wage is given to nurses for the work they do. With monetary compensation used as bait, nurses must provide written documentation of the work that they do in order to receive this compensation. Rather than be given automatic compensation for the multifaceted services they provide, nurses must submit "proof" of their worthiness in order to receive more money. This *should* automatically be addressed in terms of hourly wage or weekly compensation. Instead, it becomes a matter of who can submit the most impressively completed forms, or worse, it can sometimes degenerate into a personality contest. Many nurses view the "clinical ladder" as an insult to their intelligence.

MEDIA AND PUBLIC ABUSE OF NURSES

The setting: The waiting room, Pine Valley Hospital
The players: Dr. Joe Martin, Tad Martin, Nurse Eileen
The subject: **NURSE ABUSE**

Dr Martin, standing near the nurse's station, is engaged in conversation with his son, Tad. Nurse Eileen, with a nurse's cap affixed to her head in her off-white Television Vanilla uniform, approaches the pair, and the following conversation ensues.

Nurse Eileen: Dr. Martin?

Dr. Martin: Yes?

Nurse Eileen: Excuse me but I need to talk to you.

Dr. Martin: Certainly, ah, oh, Eileen, this is my son Tad. (Turns to Tad). Eileen is one of our best nurses.

Tad: I can see that! (Looks the nurse up and down).

Nurse Eileen: Pleased to meet you.

Tad: You, too! (Leers at her).

Dr. Martin: (Turns to nurse) What's the problem?

Nurse Eileen: It's Mr. Peterson in 309. He's complaining of chest pains. We've done EKGs (Electrocardiogram). We've monitored him but nothing shows up. I'm at a loss as to what's wrong.

Dr. Martin: Hmmm. Mrs. Quinn is on duty, isn't she?

Nurse Eileen: Yes, sir.

Dr. Martin: Why don't you consult with her. She's very good at that sort of thing. I'm not familiar with the case and it would be improper for me to advise.

Nurse Eileen: I'm sorry Dr. Martin, it's just, well, I always feel you have the answer that counts. Sorry for the interruption.

Nurse leaves. Tad Martin turns to his father.

Tad: Must be tough.

Dr. Martin: What?

Tad: Oh, being the idol of all these gorgeous young nurses!

Dr. Martin: She just asked a question, Tad. Strictly routine.

Tad: I could get used to a routine like that!

ALL MY CHILDREN
ABC-TV 1988

While hospital and nursing administrators insidiously erode the status of the nursing profession from within, the media and public abuse of the nurse contributes significantly to erosion from without. It is difficult to determine which element poses the greater threat to nursing's image, and hence the perpetuation of **NURSE ABUSE** — nurses themselves, doctors, or the media. Clearly, all play an important role. As the conversation from the television show *All My Children* illustrates, media abuse of nursing is continuing even in this present day and age. But, first, let's look briefly at the historic evolution of nursing from a public perspective, and discussing the role of the media as it affects nursing today.

The early role of nursing can be traced to the beginning of recorded history, and has always been closely linked to the art of mothering. "Innate maternalism and womanly qualities were viewed as essential characteristics of the ideal nurse" (Hughes, 1980, p. 55). Those qualities intrinsic to the ideal mother — nurturing, caregiving, gentleness and daintiness, influenced by Victorian ideologies about women — constituted in the eyes of the public all of the attributes that nurses should possess. Aggression, competitiveness and resistance to male authority were viewed as unbecoming and especially foreign to both the female and nursing role. Although the first "nurses" were considered immoral women such as prostitutes and drunks, the inception of formalized nurses' training in the late 1800s did little to elevate the job of nursing to a higher level of public admiration. Early nursing work was in a class no better than and, in fact, lower than that of a servant.

"With the establishment of training schools in the United States, the public image of the nurse underwent a slow process of change" (Hughes, 1980, p. 61). Associated as a womanly profession akin to those women of the Victorian era, public literature embodied the ideal nurse as a true example of womanhood. It is from this point on that the social perspective of nursing took on a new look — that of the impeccably neat, well-groomed, polite and pleasant young woman in a starched white uniform and cap. Pleasing in personality and intellectually inferior to the all-knowing (predominantly male) physician, the concept of the nurse-as-handmaiden was born. This was the image portrayed to the public in the early 1900s, and the image the public still holds to be true. There was little notice given to the intellectual, cognitive and educational capabilities of the nurse administering to the patient. Rather, "that she be polite, well-spoken and as strong as an ox" was considered more important.

In view of nursing's image as it has been portrayed to the pubic, it is little wonder that nurses have experienced years of stagnation in the evolution of the nursing role. Ironically, the evolution of nursing has been anything *but* stagnant. Nursing has, in fact, evolved in a number of ways. Nurses have become significantly more educated — more bachelors, masters and Ph.D. degrees fill the profession's ranks. They've become more accountable

— carriers of independent malpractice insurance. They've become more and more skilled — in terms of technological knowledge. They've become more diverse and independent in their practices — psychotherapy, midwifery — and yet, in spite of these genuine gains, they are still, according to the "public image," the mindless, sweet, sometimes over-bearing "Angels of Mercy."

The public's beliefs about the nurse's role, coupled with reinforcement by the media, have prevented the growth and understanding of what nursing really *is* and what it is that nurses really *do*. The public still believe that nurses wear caps and white uniforms. The media still portray nurses on television with all the old stereotypes intact. The public still demands a backrub and a box of tissues, not understanding that nurses may be more concerned about their irregular heartbeat, bleeding ulcer, medication dosage or their fluid and electrolyte balance than on other, less critical concerns. The media portray the nurse as the food-tray-delivery-person and bedpan-flusher, rather than as the educated, skilled, holistic caregiver that she really is.

Unfortunately, nursing practice, in the eyes of the public, has been forever linked to medical practice. It is the public's belief that the nurse is merely the extension of the physician, that the nurse dutifully acts only upon the orders mandated by the doctor. "To the detriment of the public and nursing profession alike, the public has never identified nursing care as separate and distinct from physician care" (Hughes, 1980, p. 68). "The mythical belief in the nurse's subordination to the physician, projected through the popular media, has led to the public depreciation of the role of the nurse in healthcare. Nursing care has always existed with or without physician supervision. The failure of the public to recognize this has had a damaging effect upon the growth of nurses as professional practitioners and upon the utilization of nurses to their fullest potential in healthcare" (Hughes, 1980, p. 69).

As responsible as the public-at-large is for its continued misunderstanding of the nursing image, the media is primarily responsible for "fueling the fire." At the onset of the 20th century, the media portrayed nurses as "Angels of Mercy." In the 1920s the "Nurse as Girl Friday" was in vogue. During World War II, the heroine nurse evolved. And post-war to 1965, the nursing image was synonymous to "wife and mother." In the past two-and-a-half decades, the most negative and damaging image of nursing emerged — the nurse as the sex object. Responsible for portraying nurses as sex-starved nymphomaniacs is the television and cinematic entertainment world, not to mention the greeting card companies! Since the late 1960's, the dumb-blonde bombshell nurse in a short, tight, low-cut uniform became the standard in spoofs of the profession. The nurse has commonly been seen chasing the male patient around his hospital room or chasing the physician around the hospital. If not chasing the men, then she is hopping into bed (with either the patient or the doctor). Nurses are depicted as sensual, frivolous, irresponsible and promiscuous. The primary plot in stereotypical depictions has the nurse becoming emotionally and sexually involved with her male patients. This assault on nursing's image is disgusting and inaccurate, and yet nurses continue to put up with it. One particularly offensive example is a recent made-for-television movie, turned into a regular series, The Nightingales (NBC-TV). This series (wouldn't Ms. Nightingale be appalled) depicted a group of men and women as they began their journey through nursing school. The stereotypical portrayal and misrepresentation of the "nursing class" were distressing, to say the least. Students in the school included the following: a nightclub dancer who was a former substance abuser, a male student enrolled only to meet more women, a witness to a crime relocated to another part of the country and enrolled in the nursing school, as well as a "husband-hunting hussy" who wanted to marry a doctor. As the series progressed, the depiction of, and gross injustice to nursing's image and the profession itself only continued to deteriorate. These misrepresentations lead the public to believe that just about anyone can and will become a nurse (for all the wrong reasons). It also makes the entire profession look ridiculous.

Today's stereotypes promote a negative perception of nearly two million healthcare providers — nurses. Nurse characters are presented as generally less important, less committed to their profession than physicians, and all-too-eager to enter into frivolous sexual liaisons. The nurse is almost always cast in a subordinate and usually demeaning role. She is portrayed as if she makes far fewer contributions to the patient's well-being, and as if she is incapable of autonomous judgment. In its depiction of nurses, the media makes it almost impossible to separate fact from fiction. Therefore, when a negative image is frequently repeated, it becomes "reality" in the minds of the public. Since the media do not portray nurses as healthcare providers instrumental to the patient's well being, and since they have failed to mirror the changing role of the nurse, the public lacks awareness of the many vital services that nurses actually do provide.

Given the fact that the profession of nursing serves the public, it should be a major concern to nurses just what that public thinks of them. Changes in media portrayals of nurses and nursing are both necessary and possible. Nurses must voice their opinions and work actively to change this negative media image into a vital, positive and accurate accounting of today's nursing profession. Nurses need to become more politically involved. Nurses can write letters to newspapers or magazines, or better yet, contribute to these media when the nursing image has been misrepresented or contribute to publications regarding the image and role. Nurses can lobby, protest, and refuse to watch the television/attend the movie/buy the products sold by the corporate sponsors of these outlandish media depictions that continue to blemish the nursing image. Nurses must voice their outrage at the gross injustices that are sustained as a result of persistent media exploitation. It is only then that nurses will stop the flagrant distortions that, to this date, persevere in the public consciousness with impunity.

This chapter represents our efforts in defining some of the special issues, problems and barriers confronting nurses today. Many of the abuses that we wrote about, we have experienced. In talking with many of our colleagues, it was noteworthy to us that they reported similar problems in their work settings and shared our concerns. Thus, we learned, that these problems and concerns are universal in their scope.

Many of the issues discussed here are emotional and political, but we believe they can be resolved in a constructive and rational manner. However, awareness of the specific problems must be developed first. We hope that this chapter has delineated some of the obstacles confronting our profession.

References

Ashley, J. (1981). "Power in structured misogyny: Implications for the politics of care." *Advances in Nursing Science.* Vol. III, No. III, 3-22.

Bennett, J. (1985). "AIDS epidemiology update." *American Journal of Nursing.* September, 968-971.

Cox, H. (1987). "Verbal abuse in nursing: Report of a study." *Nursing Management.* November, 47-50.

Friedman, F.B. (1982). "A nurse's guide to the care and handling of M.D.'s." *RN.* March, 39-43.

Gates, S. (1988). "On-the-job back exercises." *American Journal of Nursing.* May, 656-659.

Hughes, L. (1980). "The public image of the nurse." *Advances in Nursing Science.* Vol. II, No. ii, 55-71.

Janowski, M.J. (1988). "More from the night owls." *American Journal of Nursing.* October, 1337-1341.

Leonard, D. (1988). "What hospitals must tell you about work hazards." *RN.* February, 59-62.

Lovell, M. (1981). "Silent but perfect partners: medicine's use and abuse of women." *Advances in Nursing Science.* Vol. III, No. II, 25-39.

Reakes, J. (1981). "Nurse abuse." *Texas Nursing.* October, 8-9.

Chapter Four

Historical Perspectives on Nurse Abuse:
How It All Started

The word abuse is a painful one, almost shameful. It conjures up images of victims, perpetrators of crimes. Abuse implicates society, and forces awareness of the allowance of wrongdoing. It is accusatory. It happens and it happens to the undervalued, the vulnerable. It happens by them to each other, and to them from without. It is only in recent years that society has permitted exploration of this word, and only more recently still, consideration of the notion that abuse can be other than physical in nature. Abuse is multifaceted. Webster says that the word "abuse" means: "to put to bad or improper use; to treat without compassion and usually in a hurtful manner; to indicate one's low opinion of something; to take unfair advantage of."

Abuse has a historical dimension, for no society in any epoch has been without it. In the profession of nursing, nurses are abused — it's as simple as that. They have known abuse for the last century and have seen it in all of its manifestations. Throughout a long and glorious tradition of service toward society, the covert thread of nurse abuse and of nurses' reactions to it insinuates itself: a thread tied to nursing's origins, its mission, and the composition of its labor force.

Our Origins

Modern nursing arose from the abyss of an increasingly industrial society at the height of the Victorian era. The demise of the Roman Catholic Church in England and consequently the nursing sister orders, centuries earlier, had brought an end to any semblance of humanistic care of the sick. Home care was the accepted "system" of healthcare, and its responsibility fell to the women of the family. Institutional care of the sick was left to criminals, former patients, alcoholics and prostitutes. Nurses were, generally, "those who were too old, too weak, too drunken, too dirty, too stolid, or too bad to do anything else" (Nightingale, 1867, p. 274). Care of the sick was not a pressing social issue until the need for it became acute, and it was thrust into the English consciousness by the insanity of "the greatest organizational mismanagement recorded in history, the Crimean War" (Palmer, 1977, p. 77).

Enter Florence Nightingale, a member of the privileged class of England, a woman of intellect and education in search of a meaningful life, committed to returning to society some of the good fortune which had been bestowed upon her. Dedicated to social reform at all levels, Nightingale had studied nursing at Kaiserwerth, Germany, and obtained a position as superintendent of the Establishment for Gentlewomen During Illness, a charity hospital for governesses. The outbreak of the Crimean War gave Nightingale an arena for the practice of the ideals of her reform. It laid the foundation for the birth of modern nursing; it revolutionized the British Army as well as British society; it established the practice of nursing within a military system; it legitimized meaningful work for middle-class women outside the home; it placed nursing clearly and irrevocably under the authority of the physician; and it set the stage for abuse.

While very much the child of a forward thinking revolutionary, nursing was also a product of its time. Nightingale was a political-science genius. Even though her love of — and commitment to — nursing are evidenced in the way she led her life, that love and that commitment were definitively second to her desire for social reform. Her *goal* was success. Her *methods* set the stage for the eventual "respectability" of nursing, as well as for its feminization, its subservience, its social class distinction and its unique educational system.

In accordance with the prevailing Victorian attitudes of the time, Nightingale believed that women possessed moral superiority, and were therefore uniquely suited to the work of social reform. Consequently, women were believed to be better suited to nursing than men: "their innate sensitivity would bring warmth and reassurance to the patient, as it brought cleanliness and order to the ward" (Rosenberg, 1987, p. 217). In America, too, where healthcare reform was still in its infancy, nursing was believed to belong to the special domain of women: "Nursing is as absolutely the peculiar province of women as any branch of house-wifery. The qualities of a good nurse are vigilance, discretion, and gentleness; and these are her special qualities" (Smith, 1862, p. 149). In keeping with this attitude, Nightingale selected only women to accompany her to Scutari. Hence, nurses were and are, primarily, women.

Moral superiority and unique skills notwithstanding, women were indeed women, and relegated to second-class status in society. They were not welcome in the unique domain of men, especially in that most masculine of traditions of the military. Nightingale was well aware of this problem, and when drafting the terms of her commission, she placed nursing "clearly and unequivocally, under medical and administrative authority" (Palmer, 1983, p. 4). She knew her mission would be a failure should any other method for the organization of nurses be suggested. In spite of her concessions to the Victorian mentality concerning the status of women, and its ultimate impact on the status of nursing, Nightingale waged a constant battle. The first formal assignment of organized nursing, although sanctioned by the British people, was met with abuse and ridicule at the hands of the male military.

They were not wanted, these nurses and their services were not valued. They were women in a man's world. It was here that nursing first experienced what would become a pattern of rejection, resistance, and scorn from the masculine medical and, ultimately, hospital establishment.

Of great importance to the status of present-day nursing is the social class of its foundress. Nightingale was an aristocrat. She never viewed nurses as her equals, and believed that the only place for "ladies" in a hospital was in the role of hospital matron. Even after they had been trained, Nightingale viewed nurses as belonging to the servant class. "She established hours of work comparable to those of servants in English households, and recommended similar living conditions: small rooms with plain, simple furniture" (Palmer, 1983, p. 6). The concept of nursing as a blue-collar occupation was born.

Possibly as an outgrowth of her belief that nurses occupied the servant class, Nightingale did not establish a tradition of university-based nursing education, even though she adamantly espoused the philosophy that nurses must know the "whys" of all of their actions. Nightingale did reform nursing education — prior to her efforts there had been none. However, she was firmly convinced of the value of the hospital as a basis for training, and never wavered from this belief. (While nursing education did not enter the halls of a university during Nightingale's lifetime, she held tenaciously to her belief that the training schools should remain separate from the administration and regulation of the hospital itself. Nightingale schools were not run by hospital administrators or physicians).

Nightingale never crossed the Atlantic, but the stories of her success and methods did. Unfortunately, along with her triumphs, came the seeds of nursing's abuse as an occupation of lower middle-class, apprenticeship-trained women.

Our Mission

The service which society expects of nursing is *care*. Nursing was born of society's need for a group of individuals to assume responsibility for the care of the sick, in a time when curing was rare, and industrial society could no longer count on the female members of the family to provide this service in its entirety. While nurses and nursing were initially met with great social respect and gratitude, those feelings waned as society got on with more pressing issues. Reverby (1987, p. 1) posits that nursing's dilemma stems from "the order to care in a society that refuses to value caring." The mission of nursing and caring, historically has gained attention only when caring needs are acute.

In both the United States and Britain, the need for organized care of the sick was not recognized until the outbreak of war. The tragedy of conditions in the hospital system that existed prior to these events was not, in itself, enough to spur reform. Training schools for nurses were founded in the decade following the Civil War, and a respected occupation for women arose. As nursing became organized and its ranks swelled, it enjoyed increasing relative importance in the healthcare arena. Nurses were "angels of mercy," women with a "divine calling." Each American war improved the social image of the nurse. The Spanish-American War saw the first organized Army Nurse Corps in U.S. history, and underscored the need for caring during times of great social strife. Nurses died serving their country through caring, not fighting, and battling disease through participation in scientific research. The influenza epidemic and both World Wars again forced society to value the service nursing provided.

Perhaps if the Great Depression had not occurred, nurses would have continued to enjoy the growth in status that appeared to have been developing until that point in history. In 1920, 70 to 80 percent of all nurses worked in private-duty. Private duty nurses could practice independently and autonomously during the early part of the 20th century. Contracting their services through registries, they selected assignments in patients' homes or chose private-duty cases in the hospital setting. While the nursing literature of the day is replete with stories of economic instability, deference to "social superiors," and long, arduous workdays, nurses escaped the rigid demands imposed by institutional work. They could indeed be their own bosses.

"As freelance workers, nurses could schedule cases to suit their own needs and preferences. They could take time off to rest after a tiring stint, or take themselves off the registrar's list temporarily if sick friends or relatives needed their help. Freelance arrangements also gave nurses the opportunity to evade unappealing work situations, a prerogative they exercised freely. Private-duty nurses constantly thwarted the registrars' efforts to impose discipline and order by picking and choosing among cases the registrar offered. Doctors, nursing leaders and registrars complained bitterly about that practice. [Nurses] routinely refused certain types of cases, baldly listing their restrictions with the registrar ... an nurse could declare herself off duty if confronted with an unappealing prospect" (Melosh, 1982, p. 80).

Nurses' power to control their practice can be seen in the action taken by Chicago nurses who were registered with the West Suburban Hospital. To the satisfaction of themselves and their patients, these nurses were working 12-hour shifts. The medical board, apparently resentful of the nurses' satisfaction and control, influenced the hospital's administration to enforce a policy requiring that, "any nurse registering with the hospital accept $6.00 for a 12-hour assignment or $7.00 for a 24-hour assignment, and further, that she must be willing to accept any type of service for which she was called" (*Nurses Strike,* 1927, p. 34). The nurses found this unacceptable, both for themselves as well as their patients. They sought legal counsel and, acting upon that counsel, no nurse left her patient but, after the case was decided, the nurses declined to accept future assignments at the hospital. Panicking, the hospital's administration responded by publicizing the nurses actions as a "strike," when in fact, the nurses were simply opting to decline providing further service.

Both the rise of the hospital industry, and the economic impact of the Great Depression on the healthcare consumer, adversely affected the autonomy of the freelance nurse. The public was increasingly unable to afford the service of private-duty nursing, and functioning in an entrepreneurial fashion became impossible. Nurses found themselves in dire financial situations, and turned to their alma maters for assistance. As a result, they became dependent on the hospital structure for their very lives, as they offered their services in exchange for food and lodging. As employees, nurses were under the control and domination of a male medical and administrative hierarchy. Even as nursing leaders sought to protect nurses and the public with licensure, nurses were suffering the abuse of second-class status within a masculine, medically-oriented healthcare system.

While nurses enjoyed relative social appreciation during World War II (again, a time during which caring needs were acutely felt by the public), they were not given equal status — either in commission or salary — during their military service because of their sex. After the war, when most women returned to their roles in the private sector to "make room for their returning men," the image of nursing took a nosedive. It was during the post-war period that the image of nurses as loose women and prostitutes gained popularity — a dramatic change from the "angels of mercy" of the war years.

Our Ranks

Perhaps the most fertile field for nurse abuse exists in the reality that nursing's ranks are and always have been comprised predominantly of women. "Barriers created by restrictive and oppressive social ideologies about women have served to retard the growth of nursing as a profession, and to limit the full development of nursing's potential" (Kalish, 1978, p. 139). Nursing has long been viewed as a natural extension of woman's innate abilities, and consequently, has always been woman's work. This myth has set the stage for a history of abusive educational and service practices.

Schools of nursing arose in the United States in response to the cries of wealthy women who recognized the need for organized caregiving in hospitals. Unfortunately, unlike in the United Kingdom, financial support for the training of nurses was not forthcoming. Education in and of itself was not high on the agenda of hospitals of that era — but obtaining submissive, compliant and readily available personnel was.

This was the framework from which hospital-based nursing education originated. Cloaked under the guise of altruism, women entered "training", which more closely resembled hard labor. Consistent with the philosophy of the time, real education occurred sporadically. Since it was believed that all women were born with an innate ability to nurse, teaching them to do "what comes naturally" was wasted effort. What they did need to learn was humility subservience to the physician and their place in the institution. Nursing education was really character development, and a refinement of the socially accepted place of the woman. Nursing admission criteria reflect this. Admission to a school of nursing required that the applicant be between the ages of 25 and 35, single or widowed, and in a state of "good health." Twelve-hour days on the ward dominated the student nurses' life. The lectures were sporadic, and coincidental to the real work of the institution, that is, the work of patient care. Student nurses scrubbed floors, rolled bandages, and prepared and delivered food. They were granted one-half day per week of leisure time, and one day off to attend religious services. In her book *Ordered to Care,* Susan Reverby (1987) describes the magnitude of the abuse:

> "The danger of typhoid and scarlet fevers, pneumonia, and diphtheria could be measured in the high morbidity and mortality rates among students. Tuberculosis felled or permanently disabled many. Under the press of work, students were often re-

quired to return to service before they were completely recovered. Sick leaves were rare, and "exhaustion" was the leading reason for student withdrawals. Poor living conditions compounded the problem as nursing quarters were more barracks than homes" (Reverby, 1987, p. 64).

Women were not valued. The work of women was not valued. Education of women for the work of caring was not valued. Rather than educate women, nursing education provided the patriarchal medical care system with a virtually free, inexhaustible supply of supplicant workers.

Abuse did not end with educational content. Hospital administrations were well aware that placing nursing education under the independent control of nurses would result in chaos, and in the possible demise of the system as they knew it. As hospital hierarchies evolved, it was determined by physicians and hospital administrators alike, that nursing must remain under their control to ensure unity, as well as for the good of the hospital "family."

Attempts to educate women to become nurses in a collegiate setting opened the doors for further abuse, as nurses provided willing, albeit unknowing complicity in their continuing downward spiral to a lower status occupation. In an effort to operationalize the suggestions of the Goldmark and Brown reports (1948), which strongly recommended (among other things), that nursing education take place in institutions of higher learning, nursing leaders took action to revise and upgrade educational standards.

This attempt was met with great opposition from the nursing rank-and-file. Nurses identified strongly with their alma maters, and clung tenaciously to their educational system. Nurses themselves, so indoctrinated into a social system which valued the practical over the theoretical base for nursing believed that too much education for nurses was not only unnecessary but dangerous, and would produce a generation of nurses who "would not want to dirty their hands with the real stuff of nursing." If nursing is a natural extension of femininity, they asked, why should women be educated to do it? Furthermore, education of any kind for women was actually believed to be detrimental to a woman's health and family. Into the chaos of educational reform came the devastating, and counter-productive introduction of yet another method of nursing education — the associate degree registered nurse. Without over resolving the question of what is the one appropriate method for nursing preparation, community colleges began offering a two-year curriculum for nursing education in the 1950's. At a time when women in general were suffering great setbacks in economic and social issues, this was not surprising. With the end of World War II, those women who had been welcomed into the workplace were now being shown the door back to their homes. In order to fit the social expectation of the day, they were to marry and take care of hearth, home and children. Any education for a woman was simply to provide her with temporary entertainment prior to her assuming her true role, that of wife and mother. However, it is an indictment of nursing's leaders of the day that greater foresight was not demonstrated in deciding how these programs were to be utilized. The profession set a historical precedent by taking a step backward in the amount of education required to enter into practice. For nursing to suggest an educational preparation of two versus three years, (even though in a collegiate setting) was, in retrospect, disastrous for the status of the profession. It set the stage for the further abuse of nurses, as men and women, educated to be "technical" nurses, were utilized in practice, side by side with nurses educated for a "professional" role. Though the intent may have been one of creating two levels of caregiver, the reality was the creation of a cheaper, quickly — and less well — educated product. Nurses abused nursing, hospitals abused the nurses and the stage was set for the scorn of the public.

Conclusion

In her analysis of the society's patriarchal system, Gerda Lerner (1986) is careful to point out that while women have been subordinate to men throughout history, they did not play the role of submissive victim. The same is true of nurses. Many took radical action against their subordination, many enjoyed relative status and autonomy within the healthcare system. Nurses were at the forefront of the suffrage movement early in this century. But nurses are and have been women who do women's work in a world where women and their work are of questionable value. Our entire society is designed to overlook and devalue nurturing and caring, for it is based upon a patriarchal paradigm. The ideals of achievement and aggression, so totally unnecessary and unrelated to nursing's mission, are the stuff of success in modern society. All people in a society learn to hold in contempt those who are not valued. For at least the past two centuries, women, and consequently nurses, have filled the bill. What once was can no longer be. History cannot be rewritten, nor its value system changed. However, that which has not served humankind well, can be rethought. The exclusively masculine paradigm within which we have lived and operated — that world view which devalues more than half of society's members — and in so doing robs us all, must no longer be accepted. Only then will nurses find a place of worth in society. Only then will nurses no longer permit themselves to be abused.

References

Kalisch, P.A. & Kalisch, B.J. (1978). *The advance of American nursing.* Boston: Little, Brown and Company.

Lerner, G. (1986). *The creation of patriarchy.* New York: Oxford University Press.

Melosh, B. (1982). *The physician's hand: Work culture and conflict in American nursing.* Philadelphia: Temple University Press.

Nightingale, F. (1867). "Suggestions on the subject of providing, training and organizing nurses for the sick poor in workhouse infirmaries ...," Reprinted in Lucy R. Seymer, *Selected Writings of Florence Nightingale.* New York: Macmillan.

"Nurses strike?" (1927). *American Journal of Nursing.* January.

Palmer, I.S. (1977). *Florence Nightingale: Reformer, reactionary, researcher.* Reprinted from Nursing Research, March/April, in Pages From Nursing History, A collection of Original Articles for the Pages of Nursing Outlook, the *American Journal of Nursing and Nursing Research.* (1984). New York: American Journal of Nursing Company.

Palmer, I.S. (1983). Nightingale Revisited. Reprinted from Nursing Outlook, July/August, in Pages From Nursing History, A Collection of Original Articles for the Pages of Nursing Outlook, the *American Journal of Nursing and Nursing Research. (1984)*. New York: American Journal of Nursing Company.

Reverby, S. (1987). *Ordered to care: The dilemma of American nursing, 1850-1945*. New York: Cambridge University Press.

Rosenberg, C.E. (1987). *The care of strangers: The rise of America's hospital system*. New York: Basic Books, Inc.

Smith, S. (September 13, 1862). Female nurses in hospitals. *American Medical Times, 5.*

Chapter Five

Nurses' Perceptions of Their Hospital Experiences

This chapter is a report of a research project that studied nurses' perceptions of constraining forces in the hospital setting. The persistent and consistent constraint of nurses in a manner that prevents them from performing professional nursing practice in the hospital setting may be viewed as nurse abuse. The consistent constraint may be obstructions such as short staffing units, increasing workloads, neglecting to provide adequate backup for lunch/break/bathroom coverage, disallowing nurses any control over schedules or practice activities, treating nurses as subservient, and employing oppressive management techniques. This study sought to examine nurses' experiences in the hospital environment, and may help to bring to light to what extent nurse abuse exists.

Background of Study
The shortage of nurses in the hospital setting has been attributed to nurses leaving the hospital setting and nursing practice, the decline of school enrollments, and the presence of more complex and acutely ill patients in a hospital setting that requires more staff. This investigation

considered only those factors that contribute to nurses leaving the hospital setting. Some of the factors that lead to the exodus of nurses from the hospital setting are the (1) status inequality existing in the hospital setting among nurses, physicians and administrators; (2) difficulty of performing professional practice as an employee in a bureaucratic setting; (3) conflict of role definition of the nurse between hospital administrators and professional nurses; (4) job dissatisfaction of nurses; (5) lack of power or autonomy experienced by nurses; (6) traditional autocratic structures of hospitals; (7) insufficient value or respect for nursing as a profession, and (8) low salaries of nurses as compared to other professions.

It is assumed that the problem related to nurses practicing nursing in the hospital setting is involved with the hospital environment and the experiences of the nurse within this environment. If the hospital environment is constraining, it would prevent or impede nurses' ability to conduct their practice. It is assumed by this investigator that the more constraining an environment is, the more likely it is nurses would not be fulfilled in their role and would be more likely to leave their positions.

Study Questions
This study investigated the following questions:

1. Do nurses perceive the hospital environment as constraining in the conduct of their practice within this setting?

2. Are there specific groupings of hospital experiences that nurses perceive as constraining?

3. Is there a regional difference in nurses' perceptions of a constraining hospital environment?

Ancillary questions studied based upon the demographic information were:

1. Do staff nurses perceive the hospital environment different than managers perceive the hospital environment?

2. Does the nurse's age relate to the nurse's view of the hospital environment?

3. Do the nurse's years of experience relate to the nurse's view of the hospital environment?

4. Does the nurse's primary education relate to the nurse's view of the hospital environment?

5. Does the nurse's highest level of education relate to the nurse's view of the hospital environment?

6. Does the shift a nurse works relate to the nurse's view of the hospital setting?

7. Does the area of the nurse's specialty relate to the nurse's view of the hospital setting?

Significance

This study may give support to proposals of restructuring hospital environments (Porter-O'Grady, 1983, 1986; Styles, 1982) since it may bring to light areas of the traditional hospital settings that nurses find constraining and abusive to their practice. Any hospital restructuring attempts that may serve to decrease the constraining forces and allow nurses to more fully conduct their practice may serve to increase nurses' job satisfaction, and, most importantly, allow nurses the opportunity to provide holistic, consistent and well-coordinated quality patient care. Nurses who are happy in what they are doing and have the autonomy to conduct their practice will more likely stay in nursing.

Limitations

The limitations of this study relate to the survey methods that were used. Subjects were selected through a convenience sampling procedure. Any generalizations made are limited to the subjects who participated in this study, since a random sample was not used.

Although several mailings were conducted, a full national representation of nurses from each state (Hawaii and Alaska were excluded) was not attained. All but nine states had some representation. Other mailings have been made, and the results will be published in future publications.

Literature Review

The hospital is a bureaucratic setting in which nurses may have difficulty working. In order to understand the difficulty that nurses may experience when they work in the hospital environment, the essence of professional nursing practice was described. Additional topics related to the study and covered in this section were: the hospital as a bureaucratic setting, nursing practice in a bureaucratic setting, status distinction in the hospital setting, and administrative influences in the hospital setting.

Professional Nursing Practice

Although there are many definitions of professional nursing, one that is widely used is, "nursing is the diagnosis and treatment of human responses to health problems" (American Nurses' Association, 1980 p. 9). Human responses include such phenomena as self-care needs, comfort needs and functional needs, e.g., nutrition and rest (Hall & Allan, 1986). Professional nurses address a wide range of responses in both sick and well persons (American Nurses' Association, 1980). Nurses care for people in a holistic and humanistic manner by meeting the health needs of individuals as integrated persons. Professional nurses are guided by a humanistic philosophy which regards the individual's self-determination, independence, and choice in decision making (American Nurses' Association, 1980).

Many states have adopted a similar definition of nursing as the ANA's definition of professional nursing in nurse practice acts. For example, the State of New Jersey's Nursing Practice Act (P.L. 1947, p. 262) states that,

> [t]he practice of nursing as a registered professional nurse is defined as diagnosing and treating human responses to actual or potential physical or emotional health problems, through such services as case-finding, health teaching, health counseling, and provisions of care supportive to or restorative of life and well-being, and executing the medical regimen that is prescribed by a licensed or legally authorized physician or dentist. Diagnosing in the context of nursing practice means the identification and discrimination between physical and pyschosocial signs and symptoms essential to effective execution and management of the nursing regimen. Such diagnostic privilege is distinct from a medical diagnosis. Treating means selecting and performance of those therapeutic measures essential to the effective management and execution of the nursing regimen. Human responses means those signs and symptoms and processes which de-

note the individual's health need or reaction to an actual or potential health problem.

Professional nurses care for clients in a holistic manner and provide for the continuity of nursing care. In the hospital setting, this means that nursing care is consistent and coordinated from admission to discharge.

The Hospital As A Bureaucratic Setting

Hospital settings are often large bureaucratic institutions with their own sets of rules and obligations (McClure & Nelson, 1982; Thompson, 1982). Bureaucratic settings are organizations with a central governing structure. They are characterized by the assignment of regular activities to fixed, official units; hierarchical layers and levels of authority; written statements of administrative directives; people who are selected and assigned tasks on the basis of specialization; and policy guidance for all activities of the organization (Weber, 1960). The hospital, as a complex bureaucratic organization, must carry out its aims by defining and maintaining the structure of its operation (Drucker, 1974; Etzioni, 1975; Kanter, 1977).

A major hospital goal is to conduct business as efficiently and effectively as possible (Glennon, 1985). According to Rosenow (1983), the business of hospitals includes: 1) the availability of the service capacities potentially needed by consumers; 2) the appropriate selection of these capacities, and 3) the delivery services. The roles in the hospital setting would be that the administration assures the availability of all services potentially needed by clients, the physician selects the services to be delivered, and the nurse is expected to execute and monitor the delivery of services (Rosenow, 1983).

Professional Nursing Practice In A Bureaucratic Setting

Professional nurses are educated to practice professionally in the care of clients. Apparently, their expectations are to fulfill their professional roles when they graduate. Most nurses may conduct their professional practice as employees, since more than 80 percent of nurses are hired to carry out their professional activities by someone other than clients. Approximately 75 percent of nurses are employed in hospital settings (Joel, 1990).

Nurses as employees in bureaucratic institutions would also have a bureaucratic role to fulfill in addition to their professional role. The bureaucratic role of the nurse would be to make sure the orders and directives of others are carried out. The bureaucratic role may conflict with the nurse's professional role since the client, not the directives of others, is the central focus of nursing. Rosenow (1983) explicated that, in the bureaucratic structure, priority is given to those nursing activities valued by the physician and the hospital, and not those activities valued by patients or nurses.

There may be incongruity between nurses' professional role and the bureaucratic role (Corwin, 1961). The connections between these two roles have been discussed and researched by many (Ashley, 1973; Corwin, Taves & Haas, 1962; Glennon, 1985; Hall, 1982; Ketefian, 1985; McCloskey & McCain, 1987; Rosenow, 1983; Sorenson & Sorenson, 1974; Thompson, 1982). Some of the authors suggested that the difference between the professional and bureaucratic roles was a problem, and others did not find a conflict in these roles.

According to Corwin, Taves and Haas (1961), disillusionment of the new nurse graduate occurred since there was a conflict between bureaucratic and professional values. Sorenson and Sorenson (1974) also suggested that there was an inherent conflict between professional and bureaucratic values. These investigators studied 264 certified public accountants in bureaucratic institutions and found that low professional orientation, when accompanied with high bureaucratic orientation, was associated with high job satisfaction. However, Ketefian (1985) in a correlational study indicated that nurses experiencing both a high professional orientation and a high bureaucratic role orientation were associated with a less intense conflict in the work setting.

In a recent longitudinal study, McCloskey and McCain (1987) also contradicted the idea of an inherent conflict between professional and bureaucratic values. Their findings indicate that nurses can value both the professional and bureaucratic role as well as experience job satisfaction. However, since McClosky and McCain found that nurses over a period of a year experienced decreased satisfaction, they suggested that the problem may be related to lack of recognition and reward, and the meeting of expectations of practice within the bureaucratic setting. Glennon (1985) made similar suggestions adding that mutual respect and effective communication among nurses and administrators were necessary to allay any conflict between the bureaucratic and professional role.

Ashley (1973) suggested that the administration and physicians in the bureaucratic structure may be deliberately interfering in the nurse's professional role, in order that they may carry out their own bureaucratic and medical roles. Thompson (1982) cited the hierarchical structure of the bureaucratic setting as one of the problems relating to the conduct of professional nursing practice. Since, according to Thompson, nurses are low in the hierarchical structure, nurses then must carry out the decisions of others without the benefit of participating in the decision-making process. Thompson (1982) also posited that nurses give up control of their professional practice to follow the directives of the more powerful (physicians and administrators) in the work setting.

In 1981, Wolf claimed that four out of 10 nurses each year left the hospital setting. The rationale given for the turnover rate was nurses' false expectations of the practice setting, unreasonable practice situations, lack of support by supervisors, administrative policy and philosophy, salary and — very importantly — lack of autonomy and professional recognition. Recent reports (Agovino, 1989; Lewin, 1987) indicate that nurses still are leaving the hospital setting.

Status Distinction In The Hospital Setting
Status distinction is the differentiation of status, respect and value given to one work group over another in a particular work setting, e.g., the respect given to lawyers as opposed to law clerks. The distinction may be based on society biases, or the work setting's biases for monetary or other gain. In the hospital setting, there is an unequal status accorded to physicians and nurses, with physicians receiving the highest status (Ashley, 1973; Roberts, 1983).

The status inequality of nurses in society began with the origins of nursing. (Aiken, 1983; Ashley, 1976; Deloughery, 1977; Scoloveno, 1983; Vance, 1985). Prior to the development of training programs, nursing was an intuitive response of caring for those who were ill. This was conceived as a feminine quality or trait. Ashley (1976) described that in the hospital "[t]he role of women (nurses) was very early conceived as that caring for the 'hospital family' (p. 17)". Nurses, who resided in the hospital setting, 'nursed' the ill and looked after the physicians, often assuming all the decision-making when the physicians left the hospital and then abnegating all decision-making when they returned (Ashley, 1976).

A game that served to perpetuate status inequality was described by Stein (1965). The game consisted of nurses pretending that they were not making any decisions, or significant recommendations or contributions to patient care, and physicians pretending that all patient care decisions emanated from the all-knowing physician. According to Tanner (1990), the Doctor-Nurse game persists today. Roberts (1983) helped to shed some light on the motivation of nurses to perpetuate status inequality in her riveting article on oppressed group behavior. According to Roberts (1983), nurses are controlled by forces that have greater status, power and prestige. As a coping measure, nurses take on the tenets of the more powerful group. When nurses assimilate some of the values and norms of the dominant group (administration and physicians), they negatively value their own characteristics and contributions.

Physicians gained their status in America, for the most part, through discoveries and events outside the field of medical science. According to Bullough and Bullough (1969) and, later, Starr (1982), the technological advances in the 1940s contributed to the rise of the medical profession's status in American society. For instance, the discovery of penicillin gave physicians some power in curing disease. In addition, Starr (1982) indicated that physicians increased their status when they began to rely on one another for exchange of information and referrals. Physicians became what appeared to be a united group. Similarly, Mechanic (1983) suggested that the trend of specialization into clear, narrow fields of practice not only helped the development and learning of information related to the specialized area of knowledge, but also the physicians' dependence on one another. As the physician's knowledge and practice became more specialized, the status of the physician heightened (Mechanic, 1983).

The nurses' power and autonomy over practice within the hospital are linked to the status accorded to nurses. Bullough and Bullough (1969) and Aiken (1983) discussed the movement of graduate nurses back into the hospital setting during the Depression era and how this cost nurses the control over their practice. Aiken (1983) posited that this loss of job autonomy was closely related to societal withholding of autonomy for all women. Ashley (1973) also suggested that it was the concerted effort of both medicine and administration to decrease nurses' power through miscommunication, autocratic decision-making and coercion methods.

In line with other authors on the topic, Ellis and Hartly (1984) suggested that, in the healthcare delivery system, nurses have almost no power. Besides citing the cause as related to the fact that most nurses are women, they also suggested that it was related to a lack of knowledge of how to gain and use power.

McClure and Nelson (1982) suggested that the nurse's sense of powerlessness was most severe in interprofessional relationships with physicians. These authors described that it was the status distinction held by physicians, concerning the value of nursing's contribution to the care of the patient, as compared to that of the physicians, that prompted nurses' sense of powerlessness.

The devaluation of nursing activities by physicians was supported in a study by Webster (1985) concerning medical students' perceptions of the role of the nurse. Sixty medical students (40 males, 20 females) were surveyed from one medical school. The results indicated that the vast majority of students (67%) assumed that nursing was essentially a lower level than medicine or entirely dependent on the physician's supervision. These authors further suggested that it was "the perceived power [status] differential between medicine and nursing that appeared to be the biggest factor in the invisibility and devaluation by many medical students of the contributions nurses provided (p. 317)."

Administrative Forces

Administrative forces may take several forms, e.g., hierarchical position of the nurse, the managerial advancement of nurses without leadership experience, the amount of control of nursing's budget, and administration's value of curing over caring. As an employee, the professional nurse who is delivering care to the patient may be seen as a low person in the hierarchy. The nurse is traditionally called "staff nurse", as if the nurse performs only in an advisory capacity and not as a line worker. A line worker performs the work of the organization and has authority and power (Bernhard & Walsh, 1981). Therefore, since the work of hospitals is the delivery of patient care, nurses are line workers.

The managerial advancement of clinically experienced nurses, with no leadership education or training, to management positions, renders them unable to be effective leaders (Mottaz, 1988). They may be ineffective in gaining resources or making necessary changes as well as ineffective in supporting their nursing staff (Mottaz, 1988). In essence, they can become as oppressed as the nursing staff. The presence of powerless nurse leaders can lead to powerless nurses (Kelly, 1978).

Administration may keep a tight reign on nursing's budget, which can disable nurse leaders from hiring more nurses (Passau-Buck, 1982). When nurse leaders do not have control over the budget, they continue to be controlled by others.

When administrators view nursing as woman's work, or as less important than physicians (Ashley, 1976; Lovell, 1982), they hinder nurses in their practice. In addition, administrators who value technology and curing (medicine) over caring (nursing) (Passau-Buck, 1982) will not provide the support necessary to enable nurses to practice fully and effectively.

Nurses' ability to conduct their practice in the bureaucratic setting may be related to power, gender, status, administrative or bureaucratic issues. These influences may be constraining to nurses in their hospital practices. This study examined nurses' perceptions of the constraining forces of bureaucratic settings.

METHODOLOGY

Design of Study

This study was designed to survey nurses regarding their perceptions of experiences in the hospital environment. In addition, a demographic data form was used to gain a profile of the subjects who participated in the study.

Description of Instruments

Two instruments were used in this study: (1) The Hospital Nurse Experiences Questionnaire (HNEQ) (see Table 1) and (2) a demographic data form. Both instruments were developed by the investigator.

The Hospital Nurse Experiences Questionnaire (HNEQ)

The questionnaire was a 40 item Likert Scale form to determine what experiences nurses were having in the hospital setting. Each of the items represented an experience a nurse may have in the hospital setting. Twenty-two of the items were written in a negative fashion to reflect abusive or constraining experiences (on Table 1, see Nos. 1-8, 12, 14-17, 20, and 23-30). Eighteen of the responses were written in a positive format and represented non-abusive or non-constraining experiences (on Table 1 see Nos. 9-11, 18, 19, 21, 22 and 31-40). These 18 items were reverse scored in order to establish a meaningful score for the entire questionnaire. The experiences indicated on the HNEQ were extrapolated from the literature by the investigator.

The Likert scale on the HNEQ varied from 1 to 5 (see Table 1). One indicated strong agreement with an item on the questionnaire, 2 indicated basic agreement with item, 3 indicated uncertainty, 4 indicated disagreement, and 5 strong disagreement with item. The subjects were instructed to circle the number next to each item on the questionnaire which best reflected their hospital experiences. Since there were 40 items, a subject could receive a possible score ranging from 40 to 200 on the entire HNEQ.

The HNEQ was validated by two cont(rt experts who are leaders in nursing. The first is a nurse journalist who has written, spoken to radio and television audiences, and acted politically on the abuse of nurses. The second expert is a nurse administrator in a large metropolitan hospital. As she climbed the hierarchical ladder in a bureaucratic setting, she indicated that she was both a witness and a recipient of the constraining forces within the hospital. She has written about the phenomenon of nurse abuse.

The content validity index (CVI) of the HNEQ was estimated to be .93, which indicated that the experts strongly agreed that the questionnaire's content reflected constraining forces. The reliability was determined by Cronbach's alpha statistical testing. The reliability coefficient was .89 indicating that the nurses' answers were consistently similar or reliable across all parts of the questionnaire.

Table 1

The following items are meant to reflect experiences that nurses who work in hospitals may encounter. Please circle the number next to each statement that best matches your experiences as a hospital nurse. Circling number 1 would mean that you strongly agree that the statement matches your experience. Circling number 5 would mean that you strongly disagree that the statement matches your experience.

Legend:	1 = Strongly Agree	4 = Disagree
	2 = Agree	5 = Strongly Disagree
	3 = Unsure	

1. I am often unable to go to lunch.   1 2 3 4 5

2. I usually cannot take a morning or afternoon break.   1 2 3 4 5

3. Many times I cannot stay at lunch for the entire period.   1 2 3 4 5

4. Due to workload, I often wait long periods of time to
    go to bathroom.   1 2 3 4 5

5. I care for more than eight patients a day (more than 2
    patients a day for CCU nurses).   1 2 3 4 5

6. Many times I lift heavy patients without help.   1 2 3 4 5

7. I usually feel physically exhausted at the end of my shift.   1 2 3 4 5

8. I frequently work mandatory overtime.   1 2 3 4 5

9. I can make out my own work schedule.   1 2 3 4 5

10. I often feel as if I am doing primarily nursing activities.   1 2 3 4 5

11. Many times I feel satisfied that I rendered quality
    care to my patients.   1 2 3 4 5

12. I frequently feel other health professionals do not
    value what I do as a nurse.   1 2 3 4 5

13. I feel proud of what nurses do.   1 2 3 4 5

14. I often feel I do everyone's job but my own.   1 2 3 4 5

15. Many times I feel as if there is no hope for nursing.   1 2 3 4 5

16. I feel others make the decisions for my nursing care. 1 2 3 4 5

17. I have no control over my work schedule.   1 2 3 4 5

18. I often have time for my lunch period.   1 2 3 4 5

19. I can visit the bathroom as necessary to meet
    my personal needs.   1 2 3 4 5

20. I feel physicians dictate what nurses must do with patients.   1 2 3 4 5

21. I have plenty of help from ancillary staff, such
    as nursing assistants.   1 2 3 4 5

22. I often feel as if I am part of the healthcare team.   1 2 3 4 5

23. I feel that administration thinks that nurses are
    less important than other healthcare professionals.   1 2 3 4 5

24. Once nurses enter management, they forget
    the objectives of professional nursing practice.   1 2 3 4 5

25. Administration gets in the way of the nurse

manager's ability to help bedside nurses.   1 2 3 4 5

26. Nurses are not assertive.   1 2 3 4 5

27. Nurses do not help each other.   1 2 3 4 5

28. Nurses are underpaid for their level of responsibility.   1 2 3 4 5

29. Nurses are restricted to only following physician's orders.   1 2 3 4 5

30. The nurse manager is seen as more important than the
    bedside nurse by administration.   1 2 3 4 5

31. Nurses are able to set their own objectives of practice.   1 2 3 4 5

32. Administration views nurses as an important part of the
    healthcare team.   1 2 3 4 5

33. Nurse managers view professional nursing goals as at
    least equal to managerial goals.   1 2 3 4 5

34. Nurse managers are supported by administration in
    advancing the goals of professional nursing.   1 2 3 4 5

35. Nurses seek and make necessary changes.   1 2 3 4 5

36. Nurses usually seek support and expertise from other nurses.   1 2 3 4 5

37. I am paid enough for what I do.   1 2 3 4 5

38. I usually can take as many breaks as I need.   1 2 3 4 5

39. I frequently have a reasonable workload.   1 2 3 4 5

40. I am rarely asked to work past my shift.   1 2 3 4 5

The Demographic Data Form

The demographic data form included eight questions. The subjects were asked their age, length of time working as a RN, the shift they generally worked, their area of specialty, the state in which they worked, whether they were a staff nurse or in management, their primary RN education, and the highest degree held in nursing. The subjects either filled in the blanks, e.g., indicated the state in which they worked, or circled the most accurate answer, e.g., are you a) in management b) a staff nurse. These questions were asked to develop a profile of the subjects who participated in the study and to determine if any relationships exist between the subjects' responses on the demographic form and the HNEQ.

Procedure For Data Collection

Five thousand questionnaires were mailed to nurses in every state in the nation over a six-month period. Unfortunately, the questionnaires in some states were not received by nurses since bulk rate mail was given a low delivery priority by some post offices. A cover letter was included explaining the purpose of the study as a survey to determine hospital nurse experiences on a national level. The letter included a statement regarding the confidentiality of subjects' responses. The completion and return of the questionnaire was considered implied consent to participate in the study. A return stamped and self-addressed envelope was included in the materials.

Selection and Description of The Sample

The population of the study was registered nurses who worked in hospital settings. The sample was registered nurses from across the nation.

Lists of names of possible subjects were obtained through a national mailing list for a national seminar group and a national journal.

Of the 5,000 questionnaires distributed, 1,217 were returned by the subjects, a return rate of 24 percent. Seventy-one of these were either incomplete (entire page with missing answers or no demographic data), or not completed by an RN, therefore unusable. Included in the study were 1,146 questionnaires completed by the subjects.

Subjects responded from 39 of 48 states (Hawaii and Alaska were excluded from the study). No subjects responded from Arkansas, Iowa, Kansas, Montana, Nevada, New Mexico, South Dakota, Utah and Vermont. The majority of the subjects were from the East (68.0%). The South had 10.2 percent respondents, the Midwest had 10.8 percent and the West/Northwest had 11 percent. Table 2 shows the frequency and percent of the subjects who came from each of the four regions.

Table 2
Frequency And Percent Of Subjects By Region

Region	Number	Percent
East	768	68.0%
South	115	10.2%
Midwest	123	10.8%
West/Northwest	125	11.0%
Total	**1,131**	**100.0%**

The mean age of the subjects was approximately 34 years and the mean number of years working as an RN was approximately 9 years. Table 3 more fully describes the analysis of the subjects' age and number of years of work experience.

Table 3

Descriptive Analysis Of The Sample's Age And Work Experience

	Sample's	
	Age	Work Experience
Mean	33.88	9.42
Mode	31	10
Median	32	10
Range	43	43
Minimum	20	0
Maximum	63	43
Standard Deviation	7.766	6.855
	n = 1122	n = 1141

As can be seen on Table 4, the subjects most frequently (31.0%) worked the day shift (either 7a-3p or 8a-4p). Variable or rotation shift was the second most frequent shift (20.1%) worked. Twelve percent of the subjects worked the evening shift, 11.7% worked the night shift, 15% worked 12 hour shift days and 9.8% worked 12 hour shift nights.

Table 4

Frequency And Percent Of Sample's Shift

Shift	Number	Percent
Rotation	230	20.1%
Day	354	31.0%
Evening	141	12.3%
Night	134	11.7%
12 hr. Day	171	15.0%
12 hr. Night	112	9.8%
Total	**1,141**	**100.0%**

Sixty-two percent of the subjects worked most frequently in a critical care unit (ICU, CCU, ICU/CCU, Neuro ICU, MICU, SICU, Pediatric ICU, Burn Center, Open Heart, Cardiac ICU). Approximately 17 percent of the subjects worked in medical and/or surgical units. The other 21 percent worked in varied areas of the hospital (i.e., Maternal/ Child Health, 3%; OR/RR, 3%; Labor and Delivery, 1.5%; Emergency, 1.5%; Psychiatry, 1%; Hemodialysis, 1%). Table 5 displays the frequency and percent of subjects who work in critical care units, medical and/or surgical units or in other units.

Table 5

Frequency And Percent Of Sample's Area of Specialty

Area of Specialty	Number	Percent
Critical Care	678	62%
Medical and/or Surgical	186	17%
Other	230	21%
Total	**1,094**	**100%**

Eighty-five percent of the respondents were staff nurses and 15 percent were in management positions. Table 6 depicts the frequency and percent of the subjects who were in management or were staff nurses.

Table 6

Frequency And Percent Of Sample Who Are Managers And Staff Nurses

Position	Number	Percent
Management	155	15%
Staff	880	85%
Total	**1,034**	**100%**

In terms of the primary registered nurse education, 26.7 percent of the subjects received a diploma, 36.1 percent received an associates degree, 37.0 percent received a bachelors and .2 percent received a masters degree. The percentages of the highest degree held in nursing by the subjects were diploma, 19.3 percent; associate degree, 30.4 percent; bachelor degree 44.8 percent; and master degree, 5.6 percent. Table 7 depicts the subjects' primary RN education and the highest degree attained.

Table 7

Frequency And Percent Of Sample's Primary RN Education And Highest Degree

Primary Education	Number	Percent
Diploma	303	26.7%
Associate degree	409	36.1%
Bachelor degree	419	37.0%
Master degree	2	.2%
Total	**1,133**	**100.0%**
Highest Degree		
Diploma	218	19.3%
Associate Degree	344	30.4%
Bachelor Degree	507	44.8%
Master Degree	53	5.6%
Total	**1,131**	**100.0%**

This study is ongoing. More questionnaires have been distributed. Following editions of this book will have updated information on the demographics and results.

Data Analysis and Findings

Data analysis was conducted to answer the study questions and the ancillary questions related to the demographic information of the subjects. Descriptive analysis, consisting of means, medians, modes, range, standard deviations and percentages, was used. In addition, other statistical tests were used (e.g., chi square, factor analysis, correlations, t tests and analysis of variance) as required by the types of data being analyzed. A significance level of .05 and under was considered as an indication that the findings were not occurring by chance and were statistically significant.

Study Questions Relating To Nurses' Perceptions of Their Hospital Experiences

The first research question was: Do nurses perceive the hospital environment as constraining to the conduct of their practice? To answer this research question, descriptive analyses were conducted on the total scores of the 40 items on the questionnaire. Possible scores could vary from a 40 to a 200. The mean of the scores was 104.78. Scores were categorized as high (40-93), medium (94-146) and low (147-200). The high score category reflected experiences that were highly constraining, the medium score category reflected experiences that were moderately constraining, and the low score category reflected experiences that were not very constraining. Approximately 30 percent of the subjects placed in the high category, 67.1 percent of the subjects placed in the medium category, and 2.5 percent of the subjects fell in the low category (see Table 8). These results indicate that nurses perceive the hospital environment as constraining.

Table 8

Subjects' Scores In Frequency And Percent In Each Of The Score Categories For Entire HNEQ

Categories of Constraint

Subjects' Scores	High 40-93	Medium 94-146	Low 147-200	Total
Frequency	267	589	22	878*
Percent	30.4%	67.1%	2.5%	100%

Mean	104.78
Median	103
Mode	101
Range	123
SD	20.165

*N was lower because of missing data.

As can be seen on Table 8, approximately one-third of the scores fell in the high-constraint category, and two-thirds of the scores fell in the medium-constraint category. Few of the subjects' scores fell in the low constraint category.

To answer the second question are there specific groupings of hospital experiences which nurses perceive as constraining a factor analysis of the data was conducted to determine if there was a clustering of items into factor groupings. Eleven factor groupings were identified through statistical analysis. Table 9 depicts the items of the questionnaire that clustered into the 11 groupings. These groupings were examined for their meanings. The factor groupings were identified as 1) physical needs of the nurse, 2) management and/or administration's value and support of nursing, 3) workload of the nurse, 4) external control of nurses by others and nurses' level of power, 5) nurses' collegiality and changeability, 6) nurses' and administration/management's perspective of the nurse's role, 7) nurses' autonomy of role, 8) nurses' control of schedule, 9) quality of nursing care, 10) salary and 11) pride in work. The reliability of each factor grouping was computed using the Cronbach alpha statistical test and indicated on Table 9. A reliability of .60 and above was considered acceptable.

Table 9

Factor Analysis Groupings and Items Of The HNEQ that Clustered With Each Factor

Factor Analysis Groupings

Factor 1 - Physical Needs (Alpha .87)

1. I am often unable to go to lunch.
2. I usually cannot take a morning or afternoon break.
3. Many times I cannot stay at lunch for the entire period.
4. Due to workload, I often wait long periods of time to go to bathroom.
18. I often have time for my lunch period.
19. I can visit the bathroom as necessary to meet my personal needs.
38. I usually can take as many breaks as I need.

Factor 2 - Management/Administration Value and Support of Professional Nursing (Alpha .80)

23. I feel that administration thinks nurses are less important than other healthcare professionals.
24. Once nurses enter management, they forget the objectives of professional nursing practice.
25. Administration gets in the way of the nurse manager's ability to help bedside nurses.
30. The nurse manager is seen as more important than the bedside nurse by administration.
32. Administration views nurses as an important part of the healthcare team.
33. Nurse managers view professional nursing goals as at least equal to managerial goals.
34. Nurse managers are supported by administration in advancing the goals of professional nursing.

Factor 3 - Workload (Alpha .67)

5. I care for more than eight patients a day.
6. Many times I lift heavy patients without help.
8. I frequently work mandatory overtime.
39. I frequently have a reasonable workload.
40. I am rarely asked to work past my shift.

Factor 4 - External Control/Level of Power (Alpha .70)

12. I frequently feel other health professionals do not value what I do as a nurse.
14. I often feel I do everyone's job but my own.
15. Many times I feel as if there is no hope for nursing.
16. I feel others make the decisions for my nursing care.
20. I feel physicians dictate what nurses must do with patients.

Factor 5 - Collegiality/Change Ability (Alpha .66)

26. Nurses are not assertive.
27. Nurses do not help each other.
35. Nurses seek and make necessary changes.
36. Nurses usually seek support and expertise from other nurses.

Factor 6 - Role Perspective (Alpha .60)

21. I have plenty of help from ancillary staff, such as nursing assistants.
22. I often feel as if I am part of the healthcare team.
31. Nurses are able to set their own objectives of practice.
32. Administration views nurses as an important part of the healthcare team.
33. Nurse managers view professional nursing goals as at least equal to managerial goals.
34. Nurse managers are supported by administration in advancing the goals of professional nursing.

Factor 7 - Autonomy of Role (Alpha .57)

20. I feel physicians dictate what nurses must do with patients.
29. Nurses are restricted to only following physician's orders.
31. Nurses are able to set their own objectives of practice.

Factor 8 - Control of Schedule (Alpha .60)

9. I can make out my own work schedule.
17. I have no control over my work schedule.

Factor 9 - Quality of Nursing Care (Alpha .42)

10. I often feel as if I am doing primarily nursing activities.
11. Many times I feel satisfied that I rendered quality care to my patients.

Factor 10 - Salary (Alpha .42)

28. Nurses are underpaid for their level of responsibility.
37. I am paid enough for what I do.

Factor 11 - Pride in Work (Alpha .35)

11. Many times I feel satisfied that I rendered quality care to my patients.
13. I feel proud of what nurses do.

In order to visualize the meaning of the factor analysis, each factor was broken into high, medium and low constraint categories. The subjects, scores by percent that fell into the constraint categories of each factor grouping may be found on Table 10.

Chi square statistical testing was performed to determine if the scores in the factor groupings were significantly different from the total scores on the HNEQ. Using the chi square goodness of fit test, it was found that each factor grouping had a significant (at least at the p = .01 level) shift from the total score groupings of the HNEQ.

It appears that Factor 1 - Physical Needs (60.0%); and Factor 2 - Management and/or Administration's Value and Support of Nursing (47%) were the highest in constraining experiences (see Table 10). This means that the meeting of the nurses' physical needs and the administration/ management's value and support of professional nursing practice were two specific groupings that nurses found particularly constraining. As illustrated by the low scores in each factor grouping, the lowest constraining factor groupings were Factor 5 - Collegiality and Change-ability (25.2%); and Factor 8 - Control of Schedule (33.6%). This means that these two factors were groupings which nurses perceived as the least constraining.

Table 10

Percentage Of Scores By Constraint Category In Each Of The Factor Groupings

Factor Constraint Categories

Factor Groupings	High	Medium	Low
1. Physical	60.0%	31.5%	8.5%
2. Management Value/Support	47.0%	45.0%	7.4%
3. Workload	28.8%	54.9%	16.3%
4. External Control & Power	37.9%	53.8%	8.3%
5. Collegiality & Change	19.4%	55.4%	25.2%
6. Role Perspective	27.6%	67.7%	4.7%
7. Autonomy of Role	36.5%	50.7%	12.8%
8. Control of Schedule	25.9%	40.5%	33.6%

9. Quality of Nursing Care+	21.5%	37.7%	40.8%
10. Salary+	87.6%	11.6%	.9%
11. Pride in Work+	6.0%	37.7%	56.3%

+ Low reliability of factors

To answer the third question — Is there a regional difference in nurses' perceptions of constraining hospital experiences? — analysis of variance (ANOVA) and chi-square statistical tests were conducted. The regions were the East, South, Midwest and the West/Northwest. The ANOVA helped to determine if there was a significant difference in the means among the regions. In terms of the score received on the entire HNEQ and the region in which one worked, there was a significant difference (f= 3.892, p = .004). This means there was a regional difference in the nurses' perceptions of the hospital environment.

A cross-tabulation of regions by scores was done to help see the layout of the means and further statistical testing was conducted to determine which region had a difference in the means. For the entire HNEQ, it can be seen on Table 11, that the West/Northwest has significantly lower means (15%) falling in the high score grouping as compared to the other regions. This means that the nurses' experiences in this region were less constraining than nurses' experiences in other regions.

Table 11

Frequency And Percentage Of Subjects By Geographic Region In Score Categories Of HNEQ

Score Categories of HNEQ

Region	High 40-93	Medium 94-146	Low 147-200	Row Total
East	189	377	10	576*
	32.8%	65.5%	1.7%	100%
South	27	61	5	93*
	29.0%	65.6%	5.4%	100%
Midwest	32	66	2	100*
	32.0%	66.0%	2.0%	100%
West/	15	80	4	99*
Northwest	15.0%	81.0%	4.0%	100%

x = 15.4, df = 6, p = .025 (significant)   * N lowered because of missing data.

Ancillary Analysis: Questions Related To Demographics

To answer the first question — Do staff nurses perceive the hospital environment differently than managers perceive the environment? — a t-test was conducted to determine if there was a statistically significant difference in the means between the two groups. There were no significant differences between the two groups and their scores on the HNEQ (p = .39). However, there was a significant difference in how management and staff nurses perceived constraining experiences in two of the factor groupings. The factor groupings were Factor 1 - physical needs (p = .004), and Factor 2 - the management/administration's value and support of professional nursing (p = .038). Table 12 depicts the means and the standard deviations of the management and staff groups in Factor 1 and Factor 2.

Table 12

Means And Standard Deviations Of Management And Staff Scores In Factors 1 And 2

		Management	Staff	t	p
Factor 1	$\bar{x}$	17.5	15.4	1.41	.004
	SD	7.012	5.896		
Factor 2	$\bar{x}$	21.2	16.7	1.29	.038
	SD	5.593	4.931		

Managers had a significantly higher mean in both factors, which would indicate they had less constraining experiences in both Factor 1, which is meeting their physical needs, and Factor 2, administration's and/or management's value and support of professional nursing. Managers were better able to meet their physical needs than nurses, and managers perceived that administration/ management valued and supported professional nurses more than nurses do.

To answer the second question — Does the nurse's age relate to the nurse's view of the hospital environment? — correlational analysis was conducted. There was no relationship between the subject's age and view of the hospital environment ($r = -.01$, $p > .05$).

To answer the third question — Do the nurse's years of experience relate to the nurse's view of the hospital environment? — correlational analysis was conducted. There was no relationship between the subject's years of experience and view of the hospital environment ($r = .05$, $p > .05$).

To answer the fourth question — Does the nurse's primary education relate to the nurse's view of the hospital? — analysis of variance (ANOVA) was conducted. There was no relationship between the nurses primary education and view of the hospital environment ($p = .23$).

To answer the fifth question — Does the nurse's highest level of education relate to the nurse's view of the hospital? — analysis of variance was conducted. The ANOVA indicated that there was no relationship ($p = .23$) between the nurses primary education and view of the hospital environment using the scores on the total HNEQ. There was a significant finding with a factor grouping, however. The subjects' highest level of education significantly ($p = .01$) changed their views of hospital settings regarding Factor 2, which is administration's and/or management's value and support a of professional nursing practice. A cross-tabulation was conducted to depict the layout of the scores (see Table 13).

Table 13

Cross-tabulation Of Highest Degree Held By Factor 2 Constraint Categories

Factor 2 Constraint Categories

Degree	High	Medium	Low	Total
Diploma	97 42.9%	93 44.9%	17 8.2%	207 100%
Associate degree	168 51.9%	141 43.5%	15 4.6%	324 100%
Bachelor degree	217 45.2%	228 47.5%	35 7.3%	480 100%
Master degree	24 38.7%	25 40.0%	13 21.0%**	62 100%

$x^2 = 22.7$, df = 6, p = .0009 (significant)

As can be seen on Table 13, the subjects with a masters degree have a greater percentage (21%) of less constraining experiences in Factor 2, which is administrator's/management's value and support of professional nursing practice, than the other groups (diploma, 8.2%; associate degree, 4.6%; and bachelors degree, 7.3%).

To answer the sixth question — Does the shift a nurse works relate to the nurses view of the hospital setting? — chi square was conducted. There was no relationship (p = .35) between the shift that a nurse works and the nurse's view of the hospital environment.

To answer the seventh question — Does the area of

the nurse's specialty relate to the nurse's view of the hospital setting? — chi square was conducted. There was no relationship (p = .23) between the area of the nurse's specialty and the nurse's view of the hospital setting.

DISCUSSION OF FINDINGS

Nurses' Perceptions of The Hospital Environment

This study found that nurses perceive the hospital environment as constraining in the conduct of their practice. Thirty percent of the nurses who participated in this study perceived the hospital environment as very constraining, another 67 percent perceived the environment as moderately constraining. Very few nurses, 2.5 percent, perceived the hospital environment as not constraining to the conduct of their practice. Overwhelmingly, this study indicated that the nurses who participated perceived that they are working in constraining environments.

It should be cautioned that this study investigated nurses' perceptions of the constraining experiences in the hospital and not the actual circumstances of hospital settings. No suggestion of wrongdoing by any of our nation's hospitals was intended. The perceptions of the constraining experiences by nurses may have been influenced by expectations and standards of nurses which were outside of the purview of this study. The findings are significant in that they brings to light what the nurses perceive the hospital environment to be. These perceptions of a constraining environment need to be addressed since they may influence nurses' abilities to conduct their professional practice in the hospital environment.

The findings of this study were consistent with Ashley's (1976) findings which indicated that the hospital environment was constraining to nursing practice. The findings were also consistent with Rosenow's (1983) findings which discussed the low priority accorded to nursing activities and, thus, the lack of support and resources given to nurses. This lack of support and resources served to hinder nurses in the conduct of their practice.

When nurses work in a constraining environment, everyone may lose. The nurse may lose the opportunity to fully utilize skills and abilities, to have control over practice and to self-actualize. The hospital may lose loyal, fully motivated, effective and productive workers — and patients may lose the opportunity for a more comprehensive, holistic level of nursing care which may have improved their recovery, coping and health status. To determine specific groupings of hospital experiences that nurses perceived as constraining, a factor analysis was conducted. The factor analysis of the data from the HNEQ and the scores of the nurses who participated in this study revealed that there were 11 groupings of factors or concepts that certain items clustered around. Eight of these factors were reliable according to statistical testing using Cronbach's alpha. They were 1) physical needs of the nurse, 2) management's and/or administration's value and support of nursing, 3) workload of the of nurse, 4) external control of nurses by others and nurses' level of power, 5) nurses' collegiality and change ability, 6) nurses' and administration's/management's perspective of the nurses' role, 7) nurses' autonomy of role, and 8) nurses' control over schedule. Since eight reliable factors were found, the HNEQ can be said to be multidimensional, measuring several dimensions of what had been validated through content experts to be constraining experiences.

There were two factor groupings of hospital experiences that a high percentage of nurses in this study perceived as very constraining. The first of these groupings included experiences that hindered nurses from meeting their physical needs (60% high constraint, 31% medium constraint), e.g., not being able to eat lunch, to have an assigned break, or go to the bathroom. Maslow (1968) discussed the basic needs of mankind of which the meeting of physical needs was of primal importance to the maintenance of life itself. It may be that hospitals have created environments that are hindering nurses from meeting this basic need. The nurses in this study have to put their own basic needs on hold while trying to care for their patients' needs.

The second grouping of experiences that nurses felt was highly constraining was the value and support of professional nursing practice by administration and management (47% high constraint, 45% medium constraint). The perceptions of the nurses who participated in this study were that administration viewed nurses as being less important than other healthcare professionals and hindered nurse managers' ability to help bedside nurses. In addition, the nurses perceived that once nurse managers entered management, they forgot the objectives of nursing practice and did not perceive professional nursing goals equal to management goals. The lack of support and valuing of what nurses do constrains to nurses in the conduct of their practice.

This finding appears to support Ashley's (1973, 1978), Lovell's (1982) and Robert's (1983) positions that nurses are viewed as less worthy of value than other healthcare professionals. And if administrators do value and support nurses, it appears that they are not communicating this either by word or deed to nurses.

Two groupings in which nurses indicated a higher percentage of experiences that were not very constraining in their own experience was collegiality and changeability (25% low constraint) and control over schedule (33.6% low constraint). These two groupings had a substantial shift from the 2.5 percent low constraint that was perceived by the nurses on the total HNEQ. Nurses who participated in this study felt that nurses do help each other and seek support from each other and felt control over their schedule. However, it must be remembered that over 60 percent of the nurses felt that these two grouping were constraining, either moderately or highly. Nevertheless, it appears that some headway is being made in these two areas.

There was a regional difference in the nurses' perceptions of their experiences. Nurses in the West/Northwest region experienced less high constraint (15%) than the other three regions (South, 29%; East, 32%; and Midwest, 32%). The underlying reason for this shift is unknown. Perhaps the hospitals have a structure and climate that is somewhat less constraining to nurses. The nurses who participated in this study, from the West/Northwest region, perceived less highly constraining experiences in the hospitals in which they conduct their practice.

Ancillary Questions Regarding Demographics

There were no statistically significant relationships with any of the demographics and the scores on the HNEQ. The scores were not related to the nurse's age, position, area of specialty, years of experience, primary education, highest level of education, or shift worked.

When the factor groupings were used for analysis, there were statistically significant findings with two of the demographic items and one or two of the factor groupings. The nurse's position (either staff or management) was related to getting physical needs met and the perception of support and value of nursing by administration/management. It appears that managers had a lower percentage of high constraint and a higher percentage of low constraint in meeting the physical needs of the nurse. Managers were able to met their physical needs more than staff nurses. In addition, management also had a statistically significant lower percentage of high constraint in perceiving the value and support of professional nursing by administration and management. Managers perceived that managers and administration valued and supported professional nurses more than nurses perceived.

It was not surprising that managers and nurses would differ in their perceptions of value and support given by administration and management. This may mean that managers are not communicating their value and support of nursing to nurses clearly enough, nearly enough or consistently enough. It also may mean that nurses expect more, need more or want more support and value from administration and management for professional nursing.

The highest level of education achieved by the nurses in this study was related to perceptions of value and support demonstrated by administration and management. Nurses with masters degrees had perceived a higher percentage of low constraint in terms of administration and management's value and support of professional nursing practice than nurses with other highest level of educational preparation (diploma, associates and bachelors).

A possible reason for this may be nurses with more understanding and knowledge regarding the bureaucratic setting, leadership skills and abilities as well as more developed communication abilities, may have been able to more effectively work with administration and management. This may have led to the nurses with masters degrees, perception that administrators and managers valued and supported nurses. In addition, management and administration may value and support nurses with advanced degrees more than other nurses because of respect for the degree. It may also be possible that many of the nurses with masters degrees were in management, thereby influencing perceptions of constraining experiences because of position rather than degree.

Conclusions and Recommendations

The conclusions are based on the findings of this study and relate to the nurses who participated in this study. Overwhelmingly, nurses who participated in this study perceived that they worked in constraining and abusive hospital environments. Almost one-third of the nurses experienced high constraint and two-thirds experienced medium constraint. Only 2.5 percent of the nurses felt that they worked in low constraint environments. This is an astounding finding in light of the professional attainment issues and nursing shortage that face nurses today.

Nurses have been encouraged to obtain their BSN, be consumers of research, validate their practice activities, work collaboratively with other healthcare professionals, maintain their expertise, render holistic patient care and control their practice (American Nurses Association, 1980). All of these activities would be helpful to advance nurses' professional status. However, it seems improbable that these activities would be possible in a constraining environment. A constraining environment may not only affect nursing and patient care but the entire profession and its efforts toward advancement.

Given the type of environment in which nurses work, it is amazing that so many nurses remain in nursing and their positions and do the work that they do. Since this constraining environment may prohibit nurses from fully carrying out their professional nursing objectives, it may lead to ineffective professional nursing practice, decreased job satisfaction and lowered quality care. Every day nurses may be subjected to influences that hamper their efforts to render holistic care to patients.

Much publicity has been given to the rise in hospital starting salaries for nurses as a way to end the nursing shortage. However, when the realities of the constraining environment within the bureaucratic setting are considered, those who are brought into nursing by this enticement may leave the hospital setting. Autonomy over practice and job satisfaction are important factors, not just salary, in keeping nurses in nursing (Agovino, 1989; Lewin, 1987; Wolf, 1981).

Nurses' inability to meet some important and basic physical needs of their own seemed to be a major constraining feature of the hospital settings. Nurses generally have a high-energy job that entails physical, psychological and emotional dimensions. Without the necessary nourishment, rest and care, nurses may not be able to work to their fullest potential. If nurses try to work to their fullest potential without nourishment they may experience burnout. Burnout may lead to an emotional as well as a physical withdrawal from work. Several nurses indicated the exhaustion associated with their work in the hospital as a reason for being dissatisfied with nursing or leaving nursing (Agovino, 1989; Lewin, 1987).

Some recommendations to help nurses fulfill their physical needs include the following: 1) adequate staffing of competent personnel to cover for nurses as necessary; 2) encouragement by and commitment of management that all nurses take their assigned breaks and lunch periods; 3) a management review of staff workload to assess for feasibility of rest and nourishment; 4) clean and geographically close rest stations with bathrooms available for nurses.

Another constraining area was the lack of valuing and support by administration and management of professional nursing practice. Nurses need to be valued for the service they render in the hospital setting. Valuing nurses superficially, e.g., Nurse Of The Month Club or only on Nurse Recognition Day, can serve to dishearten and disenchant nurses. If hospital administrators reframe the view of nursing care as one of the primary purposes of their organizations, nursing may be thrust into the forefront. Nurses will feel valued when they truly are valued.

Some recommendations that may help nurses feel valued include the following: There should be: 1) nurse-physician committees on patient care; 2) nurse involvement on all levels of administration including boards of trustees; 3) nurse administrators who have an equal standing with all other departments; 4) nurse-physician panels to review any collaborative practice problems; and 5) a commitment by administration to support nursing services by a) allocating resources for adequate staffing and materials, b) giving nurses control over the budget for nurses, c) supporting a case management nursing practice with a focus on nursing, d) instituting a clinical ladder with meaningful and valued levels of nursing performance, recognition and status, e) establishing networks of nurse experts for the internal support and knowledge exchange of nurses for nurses, f) creating research lines for nurses to develop, evaluate and validate clinical nursing strategies and care, g) allowing nurses control over their work schedules, and h) enabling nurses to continue formal education by financial support, scheduling flexibility and recognition for accomplishment.

Nurses need to take an active role in removing or remediating the constraints that may face them in the hospital setting. Nurses can do this by continuing their education in nursing to gain insight into leadership roles and skills, the complexities of the bureaucratic settings, changing skills and methods, networking and gaining resources to accomplish the objectives of professional nursing practice.

Nurses need to evaluate their work setting for the actual existence, magnitude add intensity of the constraints, and the possibility of resolving the constraints. Nurses may find it helpful to examine their own expectations of the workplace and whether these expectations are reasonable. Proposals can then be presented to the administration regarding the resolutions of the constraints. Knowledge of writing and presenting a proposal as well as how to gain support within the organization are needed Nurses must be clear as to what is needed and what will be accepted by nurses.

Based upon the findings of this study, research is recommended in the following areas: 1) The replication of this study with adequate representation of all states as well as nurses from all specialty areas; 2) Individual hospital investigations to determine the constraining forces specific to that setting as the first step in resolving the areas that nurses perceive as constraining; 3) Determining whether constraining experiences can in some way be influenced or mitigated by non-constraining forces; 4) The determination if the non-constraining forces are actually liberating forces that would enhance the nurses' ability to conduct professional practice in the hospital setting; 5) Constructing validation of the HNEQ by administering this questionnaire with other questionnaires that measure concepts related to constraining forces.

The determination of constraining forces in the bureaucratic setting may be the first step toward their resolution. Hospital administrators, nurse managers and nurses need to recognize the possibility of the existence of constraining forces in their hospital, and work toward remediating them if possible. This may serve to allow nurses to more fully conduct their practice in the hospital setting, a result which may benefit nurses, the hospital and, most importantly, the patient.

Demograhic Data

The following information is to help gain a profile of the entire group of nurses who participated in this study. It will in no way be used to identify any individual.

1) Age_____   2) Length of time working as an RN _____

3) What shift do you work? _____ 4) Area of specialty_____

5) In what state do you work? _____ 6) Are you (circle one)
                                          a) in management?
                                          b) a staff nurse?

7) In which program did you get your RN?   8) Highest degree in nursing?
    a) Diploma   a) Diploma
    b) Associate degree   b) Associate degree
    c) Bachelor degree   c) Bachelor degree
    d) Master degree   d) Master degree
    e) Doctorate   e) Doctorate

Acknowledgements

The author wishes to thank Laura Gasparis RN, MA, CEN, CCRN for the funding, distribution and collection of the questionnaires. In addition, the author was greatly appreciative of Virginia G. Kottkamp MS, RNC, CNM for the enormous task of inputing the data and running the statistical analysis computer program.

References

Agovino, T. (1989, February 27). Nursing shortage: View from the floors. *Crain's New York Business*, pp. 25, 27.

American Nurses' Association. (1980). *Nursing: A social policy statement*. Kansas City, Missouri: American Nurses' Association.

Ashley, J. (1973). This I believe about power in nursing. *Nursing Outlook, 21,* 637-641.

Ashley, J. (1976). *Hospitals, paternalism, and the role of the nurse.* New York: Teachers College Press.

Bullough, V. & Bullough, B. (1969). *The emergence of modern nursing.* London: Collier-Macmillan Limited.

Bernhard, L. & Walsh, M. (1981). *Leadership: The key to professionalization of nursing.* New York: McGraw-Hill Book Company.

Corwin, R., Taves, M. & Haas, J. (1961). Professional disillusionment. *Nursing Research, 10,* 141-144.

Deloughery, G. (1977). *History and trends of professional nursing.* St. Louis: The C.V. Mosby Co.

Ellis, J. & Hartley, C. (1984). *Nursing in today's world: Challenges, issues, and trends.* Philadelphia: J.B. Lippincott Co.

Etzioni, A. (1975). *A comparative analysis of complex organizations.* New York: The Free Press.

Glennon, T. (1985). Practitioner vs. bureaucrat: Professions in conflict. *Nursing Management, 16*(3), 60,62,65.

Hall, R. (1982). The professions, employed professionals, and the professional association. In Professionalism and the Empowerment of Nursing (pp. 1-15). *Publication of the American Nurses Association, Publ # G-157.*

Joel, L. (1990, May). *Nursing in the 21st Century.* Paper presented at the College of Staten Island, New York.

Kanter, R. (1977). *Men and women of the corporation.* New York: Basic Books Inc., Publishers.

Kelly, L.Y. (1978). The power of the powerless. *Nursing Outlook, 26,* 468.

Ketefian, S. (1985). Professional and bureaucratic role conceptions and moral behavior among nurses. *Nursing Research, 34,* 248-253.

Lewin, T. (1987, July 7). Sudden nurses shortage threatens hospital care. *New York Times,* pp. A1, A19.

Lovell, M. (1982). *Daddy's little girl: The lethal effects of paternalism in nursing.* In J. Muff (Ed.), Socialization, sexism, and sterotyping: Women's issues in nursing (pp. 210-220). St. Louis: C.V. Mosby Company.

Maslow, A. (1968). *Towards a psychology of being.* New York: D. Van Nostrand Company.

Mechanic, D. (Ed.). (1983). *Handbook of health, healthcare and the health professions.* New York: The Free Press.

McCloskey, J.C. & McCain, B. (1987). Satisfaction, commitment and professionalism of newly employed nurses. *Image, 19,* 20-24.

McClure, M. & Nelson, M. J. (1982). *Trends in hospital nursing.* In L. Aiken, Nursing in the 1980's: Crisis, opportunities and challenges (pp. 59-73). Philadelphia: J.B. Lippincott Company.

Mottaz, C. (1988). Work satisfaction among hospital nurses. *Journal of the American College of Hospital Administrators, 33*(1):57-74.

Passau-Buck, S. (1982). *Caring vs. curing: The politics of healthcare.* In J. Muff (Ed.), Socialization, sexism, and sterotyping: Women's issues in nursing (pp. 203-209). St. Louis: C.V. Mosby Company.

Roberts, S. (1983). Oppressed group behavior: Implications for nursing. *Advances in Nursing Science, 5*(4):21-30.

Rosenow, A. (1983). Professional nursing practice in the bureaucratic hospital revisited. *Nursing Outlook, 31,* 34-39.

Scoloveno, M. (1981). *Problem-solving ability of senior nurses students in three programs.* Unpublished Doctoral Dissertation: Rutgers University.

Sorenson & Sorenson. (1974). The conflict of professionals in bureaucratic organizations. *Administrative Science Quarterly, 19*: 98-106.

Starr, P. (1982). *The social transformation of American medicine.* New York: Basic Books.

Stein, L. (1967). The doctor-nurse game. *Archives of General Psychiatry, 16*: 699-703.

Tanner, C. (1990, June). *Expert caring and curing in intensive care nursing.* Paper presented at American Nurses Association Convention, Boston Massachusetts.

Thompson, J. (1982). Conflicting loyalties of nurses working in bureaucratic settings. In Professionalism and the Empowerment of Nursing (pp. 27-37). Kansas City: *American Nurses' Association, Publ # G-157.*

Vance, C. (1985). An uneasy alliance: Nursing and the womens' movement. *Nursing Outlook, 33,* 281-285.

Weber, M. (1960). Bureaucracy. In Mills, C.W. (Ed.), *Images of man* (pp.149-191). New York: George Braziller.

Webster, D. (1985). Medical students' views of the role of the nurse. *Nursing Research, 34,* 313-317.

Wolf, G. (1981). Nursing turnover: Some causes and solutions. *Nursing Outlook, 29*(4), 223-226.

Chapter Six

The Psychology of Abuse

What exactly are we talking about when we use the term **"NURSE ABUSE?"**

Is it similar to child abuse? On the surface, it appears to be different. After all, doesn't child abuse have physical manifestations — bruised little bodies, broken bones, contusions, scratches, cigarette burns? And don't the victims of child abuse have a characteristic psychological profile as well? A lack of self-confidence, a distrust of adults, a propensity for lying (the better to cover their abusers' tracks), difficulty socializing, poor school performance, a sad-eyed look. No, clearly, **NURSE ABUSE** is not akin to child abuse.

Is it similar to wife abuse? Again, it seems not to be. After all, don't wives who are abused also show the physical ravages of that abuse? Broken teeth, bruises (which they conceal with makeup, glasses and clothing), shattered bones (which they may attribute to an unfortunate fall), clumps of missing hair, the list goes on. And don't they, too, have a psychological profile — oceans of self-contempt, addictive behavior, denial, depression? No, certainly **NURSE ABUSE** is not like wife abuse.

But **NURSE ABUSE** is, indeed, abuse — only its signs and symptoms are more subtle, more insidious, its incidence, more pervasive.

The abuse that nurses experience does not carry with it the typical physical landmarks that characterize those whose bodies are violated. Neither do nurses have the recognizable personality traits — the apologetic manner, the frightened demeanor, the defensive posture — by which other abuse populations are identified.

And yet, the nurse — the registered professional nurse, of whom we are speaking — is, in her daily professional life, subject to all of the mistreatment, harshness, inequities, deceptions and obloquy of other abused groups — the one glaring difference being that **NURSE ABUSE** excludes a physical component. No, nurses are not kicked down the stairs, roughed up or subject to the ravages of an out-of-control drunk or drug user — although, it must be added considering the high rate of substance abuse among physicians, the treatment the nurse is subject to may very well be influenced, at least in some cases, by those under the influence of drugs or alcohol (Slattalla, 1988, p. 3).

But, the question before us — what, specifically, is **NURSE ABUSE** all about? — is neither what differentiates abused populations nor what ties them together. It is precisely this: What exactly are the forces conspire to bring about the kind of situation in which intelligent, sensitive, motivated, well-intentioned people find themselves in positions of powerlessness, tolerating indignities and abiding behavior in other people which inevitably diminishes themselves? How does it happen that, in the case of the nurse, a job prepared for arduously, studied for intently, executed with extraordinary skill and knowledge, and lofty in its original calling, results in feelings of self-doubt, intense anger, depression and self-abnegation?

What type of person becomes a nurse — and is there something inherent in this type of person that predisposes her towards, as more than one nurse has stated it, "taking crap?" Is this what is commonly known as "the female condition," the common lot of all women, and the inevitable result of the entire human history of sexist thought and behavior — or is it endemic to only certain women, and particularly the type of woman who becomes a nurse?

Certainly, these questions demand philosophical, historical and sociological exploration. And, in fact, these disciplines have attempted, albeit inadequately, to explain such behavior. But behavior is behavior — the way we act. And feelings are feelings — the way we experience things. And, although other disciplines touch upon these phenomena, it is the field of psychology — the study of mental processes and behavior — which has attempted, most single-mindedly, to explain them.

Where does it all begin? For women — and let us not forget that 97 percent of nurses are women — it begins at the moment they are conceived. Many times, in the fantasies of their progenitors, before conception. Given the vast differences between females and males, it is understandable that the fantasy of becoming a parent to a daughter is vastly dissimilar for men and women. After all, women have been girls, daughters, sisters — females in a world which, struggling as it has, especially over the past few decades, to combat the general inequities of the past, remains largely sexist in its orientation. Men have been boys, sons, brothers — males in a world which, by and large, remains unchanged. All over the world, men are still the primary wage earners, the moving forces in industry, the occupiers of political seats of power, the pilots of airplanes, the performers of surgery. Even in the kitchen, "when a culture develops a tradition of haute cuisine — 'real' cooking ... the high chefs are almost always men" (Ortner, 1974, p. 80).

When contemplating the birth of a little girl, the traditional values have not significantly changed. In the musical *Carousel*, Billy Bigelow, in his soliloquy, fantasizes about his as-yet-unborn daughter. His words embody the still-prevailing fantasy of, not only affection, but control, which predicts the auspices, maybe the conditions, under which girls, to this day, enter the world: "My little girl, pink and white as peaches and cream is she ... My little girl gets hungry every night and she comes home to me" (Rodgers & Hammerstein, 1946). While there are many men who have had mothers and who have wives who worked outside of the home, it is still safe to say that few men imagine their daughters in positions of power, influence and independence.

For women, thinking about having a daughter is an entirely different experience. Especially for women in the '80s and '90s, many of whom have embarked on careers even before contemplating marriage or motherhood, and who are aware that more than 50 percent of the American workforce is comprised of females. For these women, most of whom have earned .65 cents or less on every $1 dollar earned by their male counterparts in the workplace, and who are keenly aware of discriminatory wage and promotion practices in universities, hospitals and industry — for this group of women, many of whom have raised their children in single-parent families, juggled domestic demands and job responsibilities unaided, sat in family courts to collect overdue child-support payments, and borne the anxiety associated with inadequate day care facilities — the prospect of having a daughter has changed dramatically. Imagine — all this even before the child is born!

After the birth, when "real life" sets in, other considerations are brought to bear on the parents whose challenge it is to now raise this daughter. While there are arguments within the psychological field as to the relative importance of each milestone of development, there has not been (until the fairly recent contributions of feminist writers, psychologists and philosophers) serious disagreement relative to the stages which infants and children negotiate their way to adulthood. Most of the formulations which preceded such thinking omitted consideration of those experiences most central to female development: affiliation and connectedness — and, by this omission, failed to achieve either an understanding of, or an appreciation of, the unique contributions which these experiences have made to societies both modern and ancient. By understanding the fact of this omission, we can begin to gain insight into adult behavior and also into the phenomenon of abuse — both the giving of it, and the acceptance of it.

This discussion is predicated on two current realities: first, the fact that at this point in our historical development, men continue to have more power, both economically and in terms of influence outside of the home (i.e. the workplace); and second, that nurses, who work primarily in male-dominated institutions, spend the largest part of their professional lives working either with, but more often *for* the men who are in power, be they doctors, administrators, or others in positions of authority.

Sigmund Freud irrevocably altered the human experience by formulating his unprecedented theories of mental life. Through his explorations and descriptions of the psychoanalytic process, he brought into public awareness the existence of the unconscious — a mysterious world of subterranean mental processes which, he demonstrated, profoundly affected human behavior. And, although critics have pointed out with some validity that Freud's frame of reference, and therefore many of his conclusions, were based on the times (late 19th and early 20th century) and place (Vienna) in which he lived — and that, because of their sexist slant and patriarchal bias, have frequently been utilized to the detriment of women, Freud's ideas continue to serve as the basis for most modern psychological theory. And his theories remain respected and utilized, even by his severest critics.

It is true that Freudian theory is completely eschewed by some feminist thinkers and also by some schools of psychology (such as the cognitive/behaviorist school). Those feminists who still continue to recognize Freud's work as having made an important contribution to psychological understanding have — rightly, in my view — taken issue with what Nancy Chodorow (1978, p. 142) calls Freud's "unexamined patriarchal assumptions, [his] own blindness, contempt of women, and misogyny; [his] claims about biology, which he was in no position to demonstrate from his own research, [and which evolved] from a patriarchal value system and [which used an] evolutionary theory to rationalize these values; [and] from his failure to deal with women at all in the major part of his writing, even when it specifically related to issues of gender."

In fact, many of Freud's followers, such as Karen Horney, Otto Rank, Alfred Adler, Erich Fromm, Melanie Klein and Carl Jung, departed in significant ways from some of Freud's theories, and interpreted important psychological milestones, such as the Oedipus complex and the role of the mother in ways that depart from his doctrine.

However, it is also true that an understanding of the early developmental stages of the human species, as postulated by Freud and his followers, has proven both provocative and illuminating — and has demonstrated that there is, indeed, a relationship between early experience (both conscious and unconscious) and adult behavior. And so the valid criticisms of Freudian theory notwithstanding, particularly as it has negatively affected both the perception and treatment of women since its inception, they do not negate the fact that Freud's contribution to our understanding of intrapsychic phenomena was towering, both in the originality of its concepts, and in the avenues it paved for future exploration of human behavior.

While it is my intention to use Freudian theory as a basis for understanding abuse in general, and **NURSE ABUSE** in particular, the important contributions of other and differing theorists will also be included, the better to present a view which is as unbiased and non-sexist as possible. In that regard, I have relied heavily on the works of feminist scholars who have, to my mind, succeeded in reinterpreting and shedding new light on psychological theory.

In the analytic view, the infant, during its long period of dependency, undergoes many developmental milestones — both physical and psychological — all having important implications for its future life. While Freud did recognize that the infant is a complex organism composed of both biological and psychological factors, influenced by the environment and social milieu into which it is born, he placed the greatest emphasis on describing what some have characterized as the "topography" of the psyche, and in trying to understand how the processes he conceptualized brought about this or that behavior. In so doing, Freud introduced revolutionary concepts (using a unique vocabulary) which were virtually unknown before he articulated them.

The *ego* was conceived of as "the major integrative institution of the personality ... its major function being continued maintenance of the organism vis-a-vis "three harsh masters" — external reality, the id, and the super-ego" (Munroe, 1955, p. 86). Functioning in many capacities such as sensory, memory, judgment and imagination, and operating according to the reality principle, the ego enables the organism to adapt to the world and mediate between the demands of this world and other demands of the psyche. The *id* is comprised of biologically determined impulses, "the reservoir of instinctual needs which press toward immediate fulfillment ... all the component sexual instincts ... [and the] instinct of aggression" (Munroe, 1955, p. 85). The *superego* is commonly known as the conscience, the mechanism by which parental and societal dictates become incorporated into the child's psyche.

Central to analytic theory is the idea of the unconscious process, the "discovery that people engaged in mental activity which affected their physical activities and feelings, but was not available to their conscious self" (Chodorow, 1978, p. 40). Because of some actual or perceived threat, or the experience of pain or frustration which is intolerable to the conscious mind, the subject (be it infant, child or adult) relegates, through the defense mechanism of repression, the unacceptable issue to the realm of the unconscious. Both the event and the process of repressing it are unknown consciously to the individual. Chodorow (1978, p. 42) says that "people use unnoticeable operations in their psychological experience of others as defenses — to cope with lack of control, ambivalence, anxiety, loss, feelings of dependence, helplessness and envy." Freud felt that repression was the result of anxiety — that anxiety signaled, even to the infant, a potential danger which the ego tries to avoid.

In addition to repression, Freud described an entire repertoire of defense mechanisms: psychological strategies which people employ to deal with anxiety, fear, grief, disappointment, excitement, the entire gamut of emotions. Among them: *introjection* (or internalization), in which a characteristic of another person is literally taken into the self (or part of the self), or the internalized quality is experienced as being part of the internal self. For example, the internalization of characteristics from a benevolent or a harshly judgmental parent; *identification,* in which attributes of another person — abilities or qualities they either admire or fear — are imitated or adopted; *projection,* in which qualities the individual possesses, are externalized or projected onto someone else (for instance, the person who accuses everyone else of being competitive, when it is really he or she who feels competitive); *reaction formation,* in which a person converts a feeling or idea into the opposite (for example, a person insists that they don't care how their boss feels about them, when, in fact, they care very much); *displacement,* in which a strong feeling (such as anger) is expressed toward an inappropriate object or person (as in the "kick the dog" phenomenon); *rationalization,* in which behavior is reinterpreted so as to seem reasonable; *regression,* in which a person reverts to infantile behavior; *denial,* in which unacceptable thoughts or feelings are put out of awareness; and *sublimation,* in which instinctual drives are redirected (for instance, the case in which rage may be channeled into productive activity).

The psychoanalytic view places great emphasis on the early years of development, postulating that infantile and early childhood experiences have far-reaching effects and, in fact, color the whole span of a person's life. While it is not possible to describe and elaborate here on the many intricate phases and stages of development which the various schools of psychology have described, the following basic description of the psychological stages of the first years of human development is intended to offer insight into the subject at hand — abuse and particularly how certain processes may lead to the kind of self-image which predisposes one toward either inviting or abiding the abusive behavior of others.

While there have been many alterations in child-caring and child-rearing arrangements over the past century, it still remains true that the mother is the primary nurturer of the human infant. If, in fact, the mother does not provide the earliest nurturing, that task is assigned to a surrogate — almost without exception, a woman.

Central to the infantile experience is dependency. It is through the uniquely intimate and dependent relationship to her/his mother that the infant's most primitive needs are met (or unmet), and that the subsequent tasks of becoming a person are undertaken. At the earliest stages, an infant is unable to distinguish between mother and self; thus, the mother acts to provide the infant with its first sense of the external world. If the infant's needs — for holding, feeding, interacting — are met, the infant develops what Erik Erickson has called "basic trust" — a sense that the environment and the people within it are benevolent and non-threatening. So critical to later development is this stage that it is considered, particularly by the psychoanalytic school, to be the foundation upon which all subsequent psychological processes are predicated.

Initially, the infant is only aware of its own needs — for being held, fed, comforted, etc. — and the mother is experienced as an extension of the self, and as a vehicle for satisfying those needs. During this stage, as the infant's needs are either gratified or thwarted by the mother and the environment, she/he experiences a variety of feelings, from contentment to frustration to discomfort to alarm. Because the infant is totally helpless, the feelings engendered at this time lead to a strong attachment to and dependence on the mother (or mother substitute). If gratification is not forthcoming, the infant experiences anxiety and begins to develop a variety of psychological mechanisms to deal with it.

It is not within the purpose or scope of this discussion to include either the multiplicity of theories or the many and various aspects of psychological development — e.g. primary narcissism, object relations, etc.

As the baby gets older, there is an awareness that the mother is not an extension of the self, but a separate individual. With this awareness begins the development of a "self" apart (from 6-12 months of age). This experience is fraught with anxiety, since she/he now has the awareness that the object which is needed may not be available. By the end of the first year, the baby has learned that people can be benevolent, harsh, loud, consistent, capricious — and the adaptive behaviors that are developed (by the baby) to deal with this world may largely determine her or his future behavior. According to the analytic school, the child's relationship with the mother predicts, or affects, all future relationships with love objects (people).

As the baby progresses through the oral phase, into the anal, and then genital phases of development, critical milestones are reached — both physically (for instance, toilet use) and psychologically (for instance, dealing with the advent of a sibling, with maternal separation, etc.). This "pre-oedipal" period is a time of intense attachment to the mother. Because the father is not generally involved in the day-to-day care of the child, he is seen as a more remote figure. "As a result, representations of the father relationship do not become so internalized and subject to ambivalence, repression ... nor are they so determining of the person's identity and sense of self" (Chodorow, 1978, p. 94).

At about the age of three or four, the child must negotiate the oedipal drama. Up to this point, both female and male children have been cared for almost exclusively by a female and they have both come to identify with many of her qualities. In addition, because she has been the person on whom they have so desperately depended, she has also inspired their most intense and passionate emotions — of rage (at being frustrated), of ambivalence (when both love and hate are evoked), of fear (at the prospect of her withholding or removing her love). And since the very acts of eating, of being held, bathed, and caressed, and even of defecating have erotic components to them (and have had since early infancy), the mother is also perceived and experienced as an erotic object — and is the focus of her child's libidinal desires (although those feelings are not interpreted by the child with adult understanding).

According to Freud, the major task of the Oedipal phase of development is to prepare for heterosexual adult relationships. During the Oedipal phase, the boy comes to see his father as a rival for his mother's love. He fantasizes doing harm to his father and then, because of the guilt this thought engenders, feels guilty and imagines that his father will retaliate (castration being a particular fear). If the Oedipal complex is successfully resolved, the little boy deals with the anxiety his thoughts arouse by eventually abandoning his erotic wishes toward his mother and repressing them (so that they are entirely out of conscious range). Finally, "the carrot of the masculine Oedipus complex is identification with his father, and the superiority of masculine identification and prerogatives over feminine (if the threat of castration is to stick)" (Chodorow, 1978, p. 94). A boy, in his attempt to gain an elusive masculine identification, often comes to define his masculinity largely in negative terms, as that which is not feminine or associated with women. There is both an internal and external aspect to this. Internally, the boy tries to reject his mother and deny his attachment to her, and the strong dependence upon her that he still feels. He also tries to deny the deep personal identification with her that has developed during his early years. He does this by repressing whatever he takes to be feminine inside himself, and, importantly, by denigrating and devaluing whatever he considers to be feminine in the outside world" (Chodorow, 1974, p. 50). "To acquire his masculine identity, the boy must both reject and deny, totally and drastically, his former dependency, attachment and identification with his mother: A boy represses those qualities he takes to be feminine inside himself, and rejects and devalues women and whatever he considers to be feminine in the social world" (Segal, 1987, p. 138).

For a girl, the Oedipal drama, which usually takes place later than the boy's, is an entirely different experience. The delay in this phase of development for girls is thought to be due to the tendency of women to identify more with daughters, causing them to separate and differentiate less. During this time, "the pre-Oedipal attachment of daughter to mother continues to be concerned with early mother-infant-relational issues. It sustains the mother-infant exclusivity, and the intensity, ambivalence and boundary confusion of the child still preoccupied with issues of dependence and individualization" (Chodorow, 1978, p. 97).

Inevitably, the little girl must change her love object from mother to father and to become oriented toward men. According to analytic theory, "the little girl's incestuous attachment to her mother ... is repressed only after she comes to realize her own lack of the superior sex organ, the penis, and, along with it, her mother's similar lack of this much-valued possession" (Segal, 1987, p. 138). She turns to her father, acknowledging the superiority of the male and her own inferior status. In addition, "when an omnipotent mother perpetuates primary love and primary identification ... a girl's father is likely to become a symbol of freedom from this dependence and merging" (Chodorow,

1978, p. 121). During this period in a girl's development, a father's role is critical — there are ways "a father can be not there enough, which leads a girl to idealize her father or men, or to endow them with immensely sadistic or punitive characteristics — or can be there too much (be possessive, seductive, or identified with the daughter), requiring her to develop defensive measures against involvement with him and with men" (Chodorow, 1978, p. 118).

It is important to mention here that modern feminists have taken issue with the concept of penis envy and have redefined it, accurately I think, as power envy — a coveting of the prerogatives of authority and influence denied to women, largely, it is clear, as a result of the early developmental phenomena described above. "The penis is a symbol of power or omnipotence, whether you have one as a sexual organ (as a male) or as a sexual object (as the child's mother 'possesses' her father's). A girl wants it for the powers which it symbolizes, and for the freedom it promises from her previous sense of dependence, and not because it is inherently and obviously better to be masculine: women do not wish to become men, but want to detach themselves from the mother and become complete, autonomous women" (Chodorow, 1978, p. 123).

To sum up: "a boy gives up his mother in order to avoid punishment, but identifies with his father because he can then gain the benefits of being the one who gives punishment, of being masculine and superior ... a girl identifies with her mother in their common feminine inferiority and in her heterosexual stance ... the fact that the child's earliest relationship is with a woman becomes exceedingly important [in] subsequent developmental periods; that women mother and men do not, is projected back by the child after gender comes to count. Women's early mothering, then, creates specific conscious and unconscious attitudes or expectations in children. Girls and boys expect and assume women's unique capacities for sacrifice, caring and mothering, and associate women with their own fears of regression and powerlessness. They fantasize more about men, and associate them with idealized virtues and growth" (Chodorow, 1978, p. 113).

To be sure, the stages which follow the Oedipus phase are highly charged and complex and also have important effects on psychological development. But, for the purposes of the subject at hand — namely, abuse — it is my intention to describe the powerful influences of maternal and paternal infant involvement which then set the stage for life-long feelings, attitudes and behavior. By appreciating the particular intimacy of the earliest affiliations, by grasping the elaborate defenses that must be constructed in the service of passing from one stage to another, and by reviewing the roots of gender identification, we can begin to see their implications.

Also of critical importance are the powerful cultural influences which come to bear upon early infant and child development. In one famous experiment, the vocal tones of both parents and other people were recorded upon seeing an infant. Consistently, infant girls (dressed in pink) were greeted with soft coos and gibberish while infant boys (dressed in blue) were spoken to in more adult, articulate ways. When the gender of the babies could not be identified because their dress was neutral, people seemed at a loss and actually asked the parent(s) what sex the baby was. The far-reaching implications of this behavior are not known, but it seems clear that girls were considered more "babyish" and "cute" while the boys seemed to inspire responses more in keeping with the adult notion of them as "little men."

What, indeed, are the implications of such early psychological and cultural conditioning? And how do they lead to women — in this case, nurses — devaluing themselves and, by so doing, tolerating the intolerable, accepting the unacceptable, and abiding the abuses which are their common lot?

In negotiating the Oedipal drama, a girl both separates herself and firmly identifies herself with her mother and by association, with all womankind. Unlike the boy who has had to deny his more feminine characteristics, the girl is able, indeed encouraged to both retain and enhance them. Now she will become the nurturing, protective, caretaking person and those will be qualities which will guarantee her the love — from men — that she both wants and needs. The entire course of female development, cultural as well as psychological, and the female child's identification with her mother predicts the continuation of roles, such as childbearing and caretaking (of both children and mates). The child believes "that any activity is more satisfying when it takes place in the context of relationships to other human beings — and even more so when it leads to the enhancement of others" (Miller, 1976, p. 53). In contrast, "the question of whether he is a giver or giving enough does not enter into a man's self-image ... they are concerned much more about 'doing'" (Miller, 1976, p. 49). Moreover, it becomes important for the male identity that certain behaviors and activities are clearly defined as masculine and therefore superior. A corollary to this belief is that women, because of their intrinsic "inferiority," are unable to participate in the "really important" tasks of society and that their contributions can, in no way, equal those of men.

For women, "identity is defined in a context of relationships ... while for men, identity precedes intimacy and generativity in the optimal cycle of human separation and attachment ... For women these tasks seem instead to be fused. Intimacy goes along with identity, as the female comes to know herself as she is known, through her relationships with others (Gilligan, 1982, p. 160). For example, the little girl learns to value most highly the affiliative aspects of her life and, by imitation, to subordinate her own wishes to those she perceives as having power — just as her mother has. Women's lives are bereft because they are the needy little girls of mothers who, inevitably, taught them to put their own needs second ... daughters unmet needs provide the well from which they give to others" (Segal, 1987, p. 139). "Since women have had to live by trying to please men, they have been conditioned to prevent men from feeling even uncomfortable ... When women suspect that they have caused men to feel unhappy or angry, they have a strong tendency to assume that they themselves are wrong" (Miller, 1976, p. 57).

The female is considered closer to nature than the male who is more closely identified with the larger culture. In addition, the roles that the female takes on as a result of her mothering (cooking, cleaning, caring for the children, etc.) are considered of a lower order on the cultural scale. In explaining female subordination, Sherry B. Ortner states (1974, p. 73) that "since it is always culture's project to subsume and transcend nature, if women were considered part of nature, then culture would find it 'natural' to subordinate them." With irony and undisguised facetiousness, Ortner states (1974, p. 73) that man, "lacking natural creative functions, must (or has the opportunity to) assert his creativity externally, 'artificially,' through the medium of technology and symbols. In so doing, he creates relatively lasting, eternal, transcendent objects, while the woman creates only perishables — human beings. Hence, the cultural reasoning seems to go [that] men are the 'natural' proprietors of religion, ritual, politics, and other realms of cultural thought and action ..."

Chodorow (1978, p. 185) explains the pervasive devaluation of women by referring to early experiences of both boys and girls: "too much mother results from the relative absence of the father and nearly exclusive maternal care provided by a woman isolated in a nuclear household. It creates men's resentment and dread of women, and their search for non-threatening, undemanding, dependent, even infantile women — women who are 'simple', and thus safe and warm." Through these same processes, men come to reject, devalue and even ridicule women and things feminine. Women's mothering produces a psychological and ideological complex in men concerning women's secondary valuation and sexual inequality. Because women are responsible for early child care and for most later socialization as well, and because fathers are more absent from the home, and finally, because the activities of men generally have been removed from the home, while those of women have remained within it, boys have difficulty in attaining a stable masculine gender role identification. Boys fantasize about and idealize their fathers and the masculine role, and society defines it as being desirable. Given that men control not only major social institutions but the very definition and constitution of society and culture, they have the power and ideological means to enforce these perceptions as more general norms, and to hold each other accountable for their enforcement. Of course, the inevitable result of emotional subordination occurs "when subordinates (i.e. women), incorporate the dominant group's conception of themselves as inferior or secondary. Such women are less able to recognize and clarify their own needs ... instead, they believe the man will somehow fulfill these needs and then are disappointed, often miserably" (Miller, 1976, p. 15).

Of course, it is because the affiliative aspect of their identities has been undervalued (for the various psychological reasons explained above) that women come to undervalue themselves. And, in more than a few cases, women who have wanted to enter "the mainstream" of society have believed that they had to imitate masculine qualities in order to be accepted. This is particularly relevant to the nurse whose very "role" in her clinical capacity embodies some of the nurturing, affiliative, feminine aspects which have been historically so devalued. One of the major contributions of the modern feminist movement has been to introduce the notion that women must now learn to *value* those qualities, to redefine both themselves and society in terms of these "strengths," and to strive, both in their personal and professional lives, to settle for nothing less than relationships and work situations which accept this redefinition. One of the great powers of nursing is in its intrinsic ability to bring humane and caring qualities to an increasingly dehumanized and unfeeling "system" of medical care. Learning how to acquire power while retaining these qualities is one of nursing's greatest challenges.

It does not require higher reasoning to conclude that little girls, indeed infant girls, are socialized and conditioned to have a devalued image of themselves — even when the development proceeds "normally" or "well." By the same token, it does not take a quantum leap of logic to conclude that a devalued self-image is the corollary of low self-esteem. And, of course, it is low self-esteem which leads to the susceptibility to abuse — for putting up with (and perhaps unconsciously inviting) behavior in others which serves to perpetuate that devaluation.

For most people, it is difficult to envision how early, even pre-verbal influences of the relatively normal variety have the power to affect adult behavior. As our cognitive processes develop and we progress through different stages of mastery over our environment, we come to rely on our intellects, our judgements, those higher centers just referred to, in order to effect decisions, make changes and find solutions. When we find ourselves in problem relationships (be they personal or professional), or in difficult situations, many of them eerily similar to ones that have gone before, we tend to ignore the similarities. And, in evaluating our situations, we tend to ignore not only the kinds of psychological processes which have brought them about, but also the powerful cultural influences which have helped to shape and reinforce them. However, it is no accident that many people repeat the same mistakes, or that the indignities they tolerate in one sphere (for instance, in a personal relationship), they find themselves tolerating in another sphere (i.e., on the job).

The "repetition compulsion" is the tendency which some people have to repeat early, painful experiences — the unconscious need, according to some theorists, to resolve, through reenactment, the earlier trauma. This can be seen clearly in the woman who chooses a man who abuses her, divorces him and finds a similar type the next time around.

There have been many theories about the "self-defeating" or "masochistic" personality. No doubt, these explorations began with Freud's pronouncement that "Anatomy is destiny!" and in his view that masochism was a key part of female destiny. Gerda Lerner (1986, p. 52), however, has called this statement "wrong, because it ... reads the distant past into the present without making allowances for changes over time. Worse, this statement has been read as a prescription for present and future: not only is anatomy destiny for women, but it should be. What Freud should have said is that the female anatomy once was destiny. That statement is accurate and historical. What once was no longer is so, and no longer must be, nor should it be so."

Horney, too, disagreed with Freud, emphasizing the

role that cultural conditioning played in the female's self-defeating experiences. Society views women as weak and helpless, Horney pointed out. It encourages them to be emotionally and economically dependent; it restricts their functioning. A personality influenced by these factors will most likely suffer from low self-esteem and feelings of powerlessness, and such a personality may tend to provoke further punishment and suffering (Shainess, 1984, p. 19).

The subject of female masochism has been challenged, both by feminists and by clinicians who have pointed to the degree to which such so-called self-punishing behavior is not, in fact, desired, but more often a function of cultural and psychological conditioning. "The ability to delay gratification and wait for rewards through effort; the capacity to put other people's needs ahead of one's own; the belief, based on past experience, and that one should have limited expectations, and the effort to avoid punishment, rejection or guilt ... the same behaviors that are defined as masochistic in women would be defined quite healthily as being sacrificial, or courageous, or as 'facing reality,' or as hard work in men" (Collins, 1985).

Irving Bieber, a contemporary analyst, places problems of power at the center of self-defeating behavior. A child's first acquaintance with power occurs in the family, and it is there that a child, who is initially weak and helpless, develops fear of the power of others. He says that the things which make the child fear authority are the triggers in any self-defeating exchange and views this self-defeating behavior as a defense mechanism that seeks to prevent or extinguish hostile aggression in others; its operating principle is that self-inflicted harm can ward off even more dangerous threats (Shainess, 1984, p. 19).

In her book, *Sweet Suffering,* Natalie Shainess (1984, p. 41) explains that the masochistic* person, "confronted [in infancy or childhood] with a powerful other, often experiences a state of ... hypno-suggestibility which causes her/him to accept whatever the other person says as correct" (Shainess, 1984, p. 41). This phenomenon begins in childhood vis-a-vis significant adults, and it is there that the self-defeating person begins to accept the premise of the other as a defensive maneuver (Shainess, 1984, p. 47). She speaks of "signals" which self-defeating people send out to the world at large: *capitulation,* "the tendency to collapse in the face of opposition"; *accommodation,* "willing to let other people call the tune"; *letting others off the hook* and underscoring their own mistakes *rushing to hand other people excuses* to justify their attacks on her, and to rationalize away her own feelings in deference to theirs; *excessive apology,* avoidance of questioning, etc. Shainess (1984, p. 54) explains that anxiety is based on experiences in childhood with significant adults, "figures who are now phantoms that insinuate themselves into people we encounter in our adult lives. [Self-defeating people] constantly respond to the present as if it were happening in the past, participating in a kind of shadow play in which people are not who they seem to be. Such women are less able to recognize and clarify their own needs, either to themselves or to men. Sometimes truly blaming the person(s) who hurt you can seem so much harder than continuing the [self-defeating] circle of self-condemnation ... [she] may seem to blame the oppressor, but she blames herself even more ... " (Shainess, 1984, p. 57).

---

* *I have chosen to use the term "self-defeating" rather than "masochistic" because the latter has been associated with the notion that such behavior grows out of the unconscious desire for suffering, a theory which has been rightfully challenged over the past few years by leading theorists.*

In speaking about the hidden cruelty in child-rearing, Alice Miller says that "all advice that pertains to raising children betrays ... the numerous, variously clothed needs of the adult. Fulfillment of those needs not only discourages the child's development, but actually prevents it ... [even] ... when the adult is honestly convinced of acting in the child's best interests. Among the adult's true motives, she mentions: "the unconscious need to pass onto others the humiliation [they] have undergone themselves; the need to find an outlet for repressed [feelings]; and the need to possess and have at one's own disposal a vital subject to manipulate; the need to idealize one's childhood and one's parents by dogmatically applying the parents' pedagogical principles to one's own children; the fear of freedom; the fear of the reappearance of what one has repressed, which one reencounters in one's child and must try to stamp out, having killed it in oneself earlier; and revenge for the pain one has suffered. Thus, when children are trained, they learn how to train others in turn. Children who are lectured learn how to lecture; if they are ridiculed, they learn how to ridicule; if humiliated, they learn how to humiliate, if their psyche is killed, they will learn how to kill — the only question is who will be killed: oneself, others, or both" (Miller, 1983, p. 98). Although Miller does not specifically use the word "abuse," it is clear that she is speaking about abusive behavior and making the point that if one is abused — or demeaned or devalued — or if she identifies herself strongly with a mother who is, she may carry within her into adulthood, not only the rage that abuse inspires, but also the tendency to experience its repetition. This repetition may take two forms: either taking abuse or inflicting it, depending upon how the experience has been processed psychologically.

While it is true that males, both in boyhood and adulthood, also experience both psychological and physical "abuse" in our society, that word is more closely associated with females — and for good reason. "Abuse of women ... is the most common and least reported crime in the United States" (Brown, 1987, p. 7). In the 1982 National Crime Survey, 91 percent of all violent crimes between spouses were victimizations of women by husbands or ex-husbands ... (Brown, 1987, p. 4). According to Angela Browne, "in this country, a woman's chances of being assaulted at home by her partner are greater than that of a police officer being assaulted on the job." Gloria Steinem (1983, p. 159) has said that "the phrase *battered women* has uncovered major, long-hidden violence. It helps us to face the fact that, statistically speaking, the most dangerous place for a woman is in her own home, not in the streets."

Sexual abuse, too, is primarily a case of female victimization, both in childhood and adulthood. Some theorists have postulated that women who are battered as adults came from homes in which they were sexually abused as children, and that they lacked "the normal adult mechanisms of self-protection" ... when it happens to them again, they see "their lack of experience with prior abuse as a major factor in their inability to comprehend and deal with the violence when it occurs" (Brown, 1987, p. 30).

Of course, in the violent act of rape, nearly 100 percent of its victims are women. While the myth that women who are raped "brought it upon themselves" is gradually disappearing, it still remains true that rape is "a constant reminder of the extent to which women are devalued, objectified and deprived of personal autonomy."

In the medical arena, women have encountered abuses simply as a function of their being female. In the mental health sphere, this is equally true. "Women who fully act out the conditioned female role are clinically viewed as neurotic ... [those] who reject or are ambivalent about the female role ... are also assured of a psychiatric label ... " (Chesler, 1972, p. 56). In a particularly chilling event of recent vintage (1987), the American Psychiatric Association, in contemplating a revision of *The Diagnostic and Statistical Manual of Mental Health Disorders* — (DSM-III), proposed a new category called Paraphilic Rapism which was described as "a persistent association, lasting a total of six months, between intense sexual arousal or desire, and acts, fantasies or other stimuli involving coercing or forcing a non-consenting person to engage in vaginal, anal or oral intercourse." If this category had been included — and it was only because of intense lobbying efforts by the committee of the Association of Women Psychiatrists (AWP), feminist groups, and other women's organizations that it was not — it would have completely removed the criminality of rape and the violence, aggression and rage toward women which underlie its act. That this revision was ever considered is a testimony to the continued contempt which many male psychiatrists feel toward women.

What *was* included in the revised edition were two new categories which label women in retrogressive, sexist, inaccurate and downright destructive ways. The first is called *Self-Defeating Personality Disorder.* According to the AWP, the criteria (for this category) included personality and behavior patterns which, for women, were culturally assigned. There was not a similar diagnosis for what they described as "the aggressive, power-driven, exploiting personality and behavior patterns fostered by the culture in men." It completely omits consideration of the woman who, by virtue of her choice to spend her energies in a domestic setting, frequently finds herself ill-equipped to enter the job market. If this woman is threatened by an abusive and economically manipulative husband (as so many are in this age of domestic violence), and is largely unprotected by the social service system, then her opting, by default, to stay in a "bad" situation, can certainly be interpreted as being self-protective, defensive, even pragmatic. If she seeks psychological counseling and is then misdiagnosed as having a self-defeating personality disorder, her best efforts at extricating herself from her situation are further sabotaged by a diagnosis which militates against employment, housing and custody prospects by labeling her as a "type" who will inevitably opt for the self-defeating option — a diagnosis that serves neither the woman nor society.

The second new category is the *Late Luteal Phase Dysphoric Disorder,* which alludes to premenstrual symptoms and mistakenly describes a physiological phenomenon in psychological terms. While it is true that the premenstrual condition may give rise to the symptoms described by the APA (emotional lability, fatigue, tension, etc.) in the same way that other physical conditions have psychological counterparts, it is also true that the psychological solution to this condition leaves the female patient in therapy with a label which, again, militates against all sorts of possibilities for the rest of her productive (and not just reproductive) life. In essence, it forces the woman so diagnosed to defend herself against this diagnosis for years after the problems of premenstrual dysphorisa have either diminished or been eliminated. In actuality, this diagnosis may reflect cultural stereotypes as opposed to valid psychological assessment. Naturally, it behooves all women to be aware of the great potential for abuse which lies so innocently behind the closed doors of their therapists' offices.

It is certainly understandable that a woman who seeks psychological counseling and is already low on the self-esteem scale would hesitate to question an "authority figure" who pronounces her as being self-defeating. Even in optimal circumstances, both women and men in such a situation do not feel confident in their own judgment. However, any woman who appreciates the vast implications which these kinds of diagnoses can have on both her current life, be it domestic or professional, and her future possibilities, would be well-advised to ask her therapist exactly what her diagnosis is, and to protest these particular categories if they are inaccurately applied to her. Failing to effect any change, she should find another therapist.

In his book *Malepractice*, the late Robert S. Mendelsohn, M.D. (1981, p.x) states that "although medical and surgical overkill are routinely inflicted on all Americans, its primary victims are women. Female patients are subjected to medical procedures that are degrading, unnecessary and often dangerous — sometimes fatally so." Asserting that "most doctors are unaware of their negative feelings toward female patients ... [their] sexist behavior [is] at the heart of the medical abuse women suffer" (Mendelsohn, 1981, p. 61). The "double standard" practiced in medicine, another variation on the theme of abuse, is well-known to most women. "It is not uncommon for a doctor to advise a male patient to 'work out' his problems in the gym or on the golf course, while a female patient with the same symptoms is likely to be given a prescription for Valium" (Mendelsohn, 1981, p. 61).

To be sure, the abuse of women (and of the girls who will become women) is not restricted to the home or to the area of psychological or medical services. Perhaps the greatest forum of institutionalized abuse belongs to the workplace and is, in fact, the prime motivation behind my exploration of **NURSE ABUSE.** As a former obstetrical nurse, I was constantly astounded, not to mention appalled, at the misogyny which I both experienced and observed in the clinical setting. It is interesting to note that the word itself, *misogyny* (which is derived from the Greek), means literally: *miso* — to hate, and *gyny* (as in gynecologist) — woman. According to economist Sylvia Ann Hewlett (1986, p. 83), "gender seems to be a more powerful handicap than race in the labor market. Despite the enormous expansion of the female labor force in recent years — the number of women working has [more than] doubled since 1960 — there has been little improvement in women's economic position ... only 7 percent of employed women in America work in managerial positions." It is a sad commentary on the continued devaluation of women and of the importance they play in the nation's economy that, although three-quarters of the nation's working women have school-age children and half have children less than a year old, the United States continues to be "the only industrialized country that has no statutory maternity leave. One hundred and seventeen countries (including every industrial nation and many developing countries) guarantee a woman ... leave from employment for childbirth, job protection while she is on leave, and the provision of a cash benefit to replace all or most of her earnings" (Hewlett, 1986, p. 71).

In the vital area of day care, problems of inadequate legislation, of meager funding, of poor regulation and of underpaid staff workers, abound. And, although children are parented by two parents (although increasing numbers live with only one parent — overwhelmingly, the mother), the responsibility for child care — crucial to the working woman's consideration — is, again, almost exclusively relegated to the woman's domain.

Concerns as to the psychological effects of day care on children less than one year of age, on toddlers, on older children and on the mothers who must juggle parental and economic responsibilities — all pose serious questions. And, questions as to what our legislators are doing to bring about a day care system which safeguards the promise of our country — its children — remain open to critical investigation.

   According to the Labor Department, only 11 percent of United States companies provide some child care services to their employees, but only 2 percent actually sponsor day care centers, and only 3 percent provide financial assistance for child care. As late as 1985, about 1,800 employers, out of a total of 6 million businesses in the U.S., provided child-care assistance. It is not surprising that, in a May 1988 Census Bureau report, it was reported that the inability to find a baby sitter disrupted the jobs of about 450,000 women nationally each month. And, to compound the problem, although "working wives do less housework than homemakers ... they still do the vast bulk of what needs to be done. Even if a husband is unemployed, he does much less housework than a wife who puts in a 40-hour week. This is the case even among couples who profess egalitarian social ideals. While husbands might say they *should* share responsibility, when they break it down to time actually spent and chores actually done, the idea of shared responsibility turns out to be a myth" (Blumstein, 1983, p. 145).

   On the job, the catalogue of inequities which exist for women is filled with topics such as wages consistently lower than their male counterparts earn; discrimination in promotional policies; horizontal, not upward, mobility; and the difficulty, again, in dealing with those in power, most of whom are men.

   In 1988, the term "sexual harassment" has become synonymous with women. It is interesting that among the synonyms used by *Webster's Dictionary* to describe harassment are badger, pester, plague and torment. Certainly, they can all be subsumed under the category of abuse. The woman who is sexually harassed is on the receiving end of "leering, pinching, patting, repeated comments, subtle suggestions of a sexual nature and pressure for dates. It can also take the form of actual or attempted rape." Women who are sexually harassed find themselves in the classic double-bind: if they capitulate, they are filled with self-contempt; if they resist, they find themselves the victims of work-related reprisals. "These can include escalation of harassment; poor work assignments; sabotaging of projects; denial of raises, benefits or promotions; and sometimes the loss of the job, with only a poor reference to show for it" (*The New Our Bodies*, 1984, p. 108).

In the world of nursing, both job-related and sexual harassment are well-known phenomena. Be they interns, residents or attending physicians, the doctors who perpetrate this kind of harassment are elaborating on behaviors which characterize the nurse/doctor relationship in general. As a microcosm of society at large, this relationship perpetuates the role of male as dominant, female as subordinate. For those who protest that "times have changed," it would be instructive to review the fierce opposition doctors have waged against the nurses who have sought legislation to expand the nursing role in caring for nursing-home patients or who have proposed the creation of an alternative to health-maintenance organizations (HMOs) in community nursing organizations (CNOs). At a July 1988 convention of the American Medical Association, doctors, reacting to the "nursing crisis," proposed a "new class of workers" called registered care technicians (RCTs). "The AMA acknowledged that one goal of creating RCTs was to draw in more male workers who otherwise wouldn't be attracted to nursing" (Dentzer, 1988).

With few avenues to redress their grievances, the anger that nurses feel is negotiated through the defense mechanisms learned at an earlier stage of development. The nurse may use 'displacement' to target her rage onto a fellow nurse. Angry at herself for capitulating to unreasonable demands, she may use "projection" to express the contempt she feels toward herself onto an innocent patient who happens to be "cooperating." She may "identify" with her oppressor and find herself oppressing others. She may "rationalize" her behavior in order to recapture her sense of self-esteem. Or, of course, she may become appropriately angry — and suffer the consequences! Among the many psychologically battering consequences that are foisted on women are: "Assuming the right to control women's behavior; devaluing her opinions, feelings and accomplishments; yelling, threatening, withdrawing into angry silence when displeased; making the woman afraid of 'setting him off'; switching from charm to rage without warning; making her feel inadequate or confused (Forward, 1986, p. 132).

Although most nurses are grown women, the messages they (and other women) receive in childhood are that the "disparity between accomplishments for which boys are admired and those for which girls are admired is that while girls are praised for manners and appearance, boys are more often praised for academic achievement and physical strength. Girls may also be discouraged from exploring and mastering life, and encouraged instead to develop skills to manipulate others to negotiate in the world for them. What these girls are getting are lessons in learned helplessness" (Forward, 1986, p. 133). They learn that "you are good to the degree that you give men what they want and follow the rules that they have laid down for you. You sacrifice your own personal satisfaction in return for being told how nice and sweet you are by the men whose approval you are seeking ... this is no substitute for meeting your own needs. The inevitable consequence is a continual low-level anger that flares up periodically in unexplainable outbursts ... " (Fezler, 1985, p.

xii). "For most women, there is an enormous gap between their childhood conditioning and the process necessary to achieve growth and personal fulfillment ... tremendous conflict between the conscious needs of the '80s and the subconscious messages received in early childhood ..." (Dworkin, 1974, p. 23). "The nature of women's oppression is unique: women are oppressed as women, regardless of class or race; some women have access to wealth, but that wealth does not signify power; women are to be found everywhere, but own or control no appreciable territory; ... women have little sense of dignity or self-respect or strength, since those qualities are directly related to a sense of manhood. When ... women find the courage to defend themselves, to take a stand against ... abuse, they are violating every notion of womanhood they have ever been taught" (Machiavelli, 1952).

And so, the nature of abuse — both giving it and taking it — can be found in the seeds of our very earliest development, first in the fantasies of those who, before we are born, imagine what we will be like, and then in the realities of our individual life experiences. That the female experience is vastly different from the male's, and that those differences affect every subsequent aspect of women's lives is indisputable. That nurses, occupying, as they do, a profession historically associated with female exclusivity, have been subject to abuse, should come as no surprise. That the "caretaker" function of nurses evokes so keenly the ambivalent or negative reactions of many of their co-workers, both male and female, can only be understood by viewing this reenactment of ancient and highly-charged relationships in its proper psychological context.

Without alluding to gender, Niccolo Machiavelli (1952), in *The Prince,* captures the primary emotional operating principles which prevail even now, in the personal and professional lives of women and men in the 1900s and beyond. "The Question [arises] whether it is better to be loved rather than feared, or feared rather than loved. It might perhaps be answered that we should wish to be both; but since love and fear can hardly exist together, if we must choose between them, it is far safer to be feared than loved."

Must women — must nurses — continue to fear, both their own potential for power and the obstacles which confront them? Must they continue to be abused? I think not. But that is fodder for another discussion — let us call it "Solutions."

References

Blumstein, Philip, Schwartz & Pepper. (1983). *American couples: Money, work and sex.* New York: William Morrow.

Boston Women's Health Book Collective: *The new our bodies, ourselves.* (1984). New York: Simon & Schuster.

Brown, Angela. (1987). *When battered women kill.* New York: Free Press/MacMillan.

Chesler, Phillis. (1972). *Women and madness.* New York: Avon Books.

Chodorow, Nancy. (1974). Family structure and feminine personality, in *Women culture and society.* Rosaldo, M. and Lamphere, L. (eds). Stanford: Stanford University Press.

Chodorow, Nancy. (1978). *"The reproduction of mothering": Psychoanalysis and the sociology of gender.* California: University of California Press.

Collins, Glenn. *New York Times.* "Women & masochism: Debate continues." (1985). (Interview with Dr. Paula Caplan). New York, New York. December 12, 1985.

Dentzer, Susan. (1988). "Calling the shots in health care: The nursing shortage points up a growing turf war between doctors and nurses." *U.S. News and World Report.* July 11.

Dworkin, Andrea. (1974). *Woman hating.* New York: E.P. Dutton.

Fezler, William & Field, Eleanor Ph.D. (1985). *The good girl syndrome.* New York: MacMillan, (preface).

Forward, Dr. Susan and Torres, Joan. (1986). *Men who hate women and the women who love them.* New York: Bantam Books.

Gilligan, Carl. (1982). *In a different voice: Psychological theory and women's development.* Cambridge: Harvard University Press.

Hewlett, Sylvia Ann. (1986). *A lesser life: The myth of women's liberation in America.* New York: Warner Books.

Lerner, Gerda. (1986). *The creation of patriarchy.* New York: Oxford University Press.

Machiavelli, Niccolo. (1952). *The prince.* New York: New American Library.

Mendelsohn, Robert S. M.D. (1981). *Malepractice: How doctors manipulate women.* Chicago: Contemporary Books, Inc.

Miller, Alice. (1983). *Hidden cruelty in child-rearing and the roots of violence.* New York: Farrar, Straus, Giroux.

Miller, Jean Baker. (1976). *Toward a new psychology of women.* Boston: Beacon Press.

Munroe, Ruth L. (1955). *Schools of psychodynamic thought.* New York: The Dryden Press Publishers.

Ortner, Sherry B. (1974). "Is female is to male as nature is to culture?", in *Woman, culture and society.* Rosaldo, M. and L. Lamphere., (eds.), Stanford: Stanford University Press.

Rodgers, Richard & Hammerstein II, Oscar. (1946). *Carousel.* copyright Chappell Music Publishing Co.

Segal, Lynne. (1987). *Is the future female: Troubled thoughts on contemporary feminism.* New York: Peter Bedrick Press.

Shainess, Natalie. (1984). *Sweet suffering.* Indianapolis/New York: Bobbs-Merrill Company, Inc.

Slattalla, Michelle. (1988). *Newsday.* Help for addicted M.D.s called lax.   Long Island, New York, March 6.

Steinem, Gloria. (1983). *Outrageous acts and everyday rebellions.* New York: Holt, Rhinehart & Winston.

Chapter Seven

Another Look At Burnout

Few will deny that nursing is a stressful occupation. The demands made on nurses are considered excessive by many. It seems logical, then, that if the stress placed on nurses continues undiminished and without relief, burnout is bound to occur.

Professional burnout, as defined in the cumulative Index of Nursing and Allied Health Literature, 1987, is "An excessive stress reaction to one's occupational or professional environment. It is manifested by feelings of emotional and physical exhaustion coupled with a sense of frustration and failure." Cherniss (1987, p. 55) describes burnout simply as "negative changes in work related attitudes and behavior in response to job stress" He elaborates by defining burnout to include " increasing discouragement, pessimism and fatalism about one's work; decline in motivation, effort and involvement in work; apathy; negativism; frequent irritability and anger with clients and colleagues;" ... "resistance to change, growing rigidity and loss of creativity" (Firth, 1986, p. 634). My own definition of burnout is based on my personal experience as a nurse and would be "a depressed or apathetic state on the part of the caretaker due to unreasonably high ex-

212 NURSE ABUSE: IMPACT AND RESOLUTION

pectations of both quantity and quality of care, in an unreasonably short period of time."

What happens, then, to the enthusiasm, excitement
and sense of caring that the new nurse brings to her work
setting? Obviously, the pressures, stresses and traumas
that occur (some more subtle than others) bring about this
sad but all-too-common transformation from supercharged
novice to burned-out veteran.

This chapter will discuss some of the situations in
which nurses find themselves, many of which may lead to
burnout.

Nurses in the hospital setting are set up to fail.
Typically, they learn to complete a large volume of complex work in a very short period of time. However, regardless of the degree of work completed, someone is always
quick to point out the part of the job that was overlooked.
Nurses do not receive a great deal of positive reinforcement. Frustration results from doing one's best, and finding that only the work left undone is remarked upon.

The problem in healthcare agencies is that there are
real differences in goals, and these differences lead to major conflicts. "Inflation and fiscal constraints are forcing
nurse managers to promote cost containment in the face
of professional desires to maintain high quality of service,
and of personal needs to maintain high quality of service,
and of personal needs to protect one's own standard of living" (Levenstein, 1980, p. 47). Therefore, nurses are torn
between their loyalty to their profession or their employing
institutions.

What are the reasons for the gap between nurses'
needs and goals and those of the hospital administrations?
One is that hospital nursing has changed dramatically
over the past several years. Due to the advent of DRGs
(Diagnostic Related Groups) patients' rates of stay have
shortened considerably. At the same time, the sophistica-

tion and awareness of hospitalized patients have risen dramatically and, with it, a concomitant expectation that nurses increase their knowledge of both medicine and technology. Nurses must now utilize various types of controllers and pumps, recognize lethal arrhythmias and know their treatments, be able to "troubleshoot" respirators and other machinery, and have a good working knowledge of medicine in order to work as members of a team with doctors. They must be prepared to assist with complex surgical procedures, administer medications safely, understand the dietary needs of their patients, and teach their patients about their diagnoses, treatments, medications, etc. The list of responsibilities seems to be endless.

More seriously ill patients are surviving, which has made the nurse's work even more physically taxing. It is not uncommon, for example, to find patients in their eighties and nineties with multiple organ failure being treated aggressively. A common example is the patient whose lungs have failed and is being maintained on a respirator. He now requires a tremendous number of nursing care hours since he is unable to perform any activities of daily living himself. He must be bathed at least daily, and care must be taken to keep his airway patent by frequent suctioning. His medications and feedings must be given through a tube to his stomach, and intravenous fluids and medications must be monitored continuously. Meticulous skin care must be rendered, including turning the patient on a regular and frequent basis, and massaging his skin to prevent bed sores. One official of the Department of Health and Human Services predicts that "hospitals will be huge intensive care units by the 1990s" (Aiken, 1982, p. 66).

The result is that nursing has become more stressful than ever before. The term "holistic care," currently in common use, means that nurses must care for every need of their patients — physical, psychological, emotional and psychosocial. Our job descriptions include much more than "the promotion and restoration of health, the prevention of illness, and the alleviation of suffering" (Bullough, 1983, p. 69). We are also mothers/fathers, psychologists, social workers, technicians for complex machinery, and confidants to our patients and/or their families.

A Typical Day for a Nurse on a Medical-Surgical Floor

Because of the increased number of responsibilities, nurses must function in an extremely organized manner if they hope to complete their work within the limits of an eight-or-12-hour shift. The shift usually begins with a narcotic count by two nurses. Then report is begun. If the shift is from 7 a.m.- 3:30 p.m., report should be finished by 7:45 a.m. Report is a detailed synopsis of each patient, including diagnosis, tests already completed and their results, exams which are planned in the immediate future, blood value results, intravenous solutions being administered, and the overall current status of the patient, including any unusual occurrences, i.e., chest pain, vomiting, etc.

Then the nurse begins taking vital signs, which includes assessing and charting the patient's temperature, pulse, respirations and blood pressure. Bed baths usually follow, during which time the nurse evaluates her patient's skin, listens to his lungs by auscultation, checks his response to medications for adverse reactions, evaluates his tolerance of feedings, assesses the patient's orientation to time, place and person, and interprets the tracings on the cardiac monitor if one is at the bedside. Bedmaking is usually done at this time — often not an easy task, if the patient is bedridden and/or comatose. Many patients must be fed, usually a slow and time-consuming process. If they are fed via a nasogastric tube (going through the nose to the stomach), the tube must be checked for placement and potency prior to placing new feeding in progress. Other patients are fed intravenously only, and even greater care is taken with this solution (known as hyperalimentation), since these patients must be weighed daily and must have their blood sugar level checked every four to six hours. Nine a.m. medications will be distributed by approximately 10:15 a.m.; medication distribution is not a simple matter of giving out some pills — it includes maintenance of intravenous fluids at the proper rate, administering antibiotics intravenously, and giving pills orally as well as through feeding tubes. Some routine medications must be given by injection, and still others must not be given until the patient's blood pressure and pulse are known, since they may only be given when these vital signs are within a certain range. The nurse then, does not give medications blindly by order from the physician, but she must be aware of the effects, side effects, contraindications of these medications and recognize allergic reactions. She must also be familiar with the normal dosages of all medications so as to question an unusual order. The nurse may spend a great deal of time paging physicians in this endeavor.

Following the medication administration, certain procedures and regimens must be performed for the patients. These include tracheal suctioning, or removal of mucus from a patient's airway so that he/she can breathe comfortably, turning the immobile patient from side to side every two hours so that bedsores will not develop, massaging the skin and performing passive exercises of the patient's joints to prevent him/her from becoming extremely stiff. Intravenous bags must be replaced before they are empty.

Patients' conditions are often unstable, and therefore the shift may be completely unpredictable in terms of the care that will be indicated. Patients may complain of chest pain. They may have difficulty breathing, exhibit heavy bleeding, require blood transfusions, or need pre-operative teaching. If surgery is scheduled, the nurse must complete the chart so that the patient is cleared for surgery.

Now it is noon, the vital signs again must be taken for unstable patients. Noon, 1 p.m. and 2 p.m., medications must be given and patients must be fed lunch. Then there are bedpans, changing incontinent patients, and notes to be written on every patient. Now, if all "goes well," the nurse may get a break, possibly even a lunch hour. That's assuming, of course, that everything runs smoothly and the patients remain stable. (Never assume — due to the larger number of elderly patients with multiple organ failure, it is rare that all assigned patients remain stable.)

I would like to relate a story which demonstrates a typical problem with which a nurse might be confronted. While I was working as a clinical instructor one day, a student was completing a pre-operative checklist. We spent at least an hour straightening out all the problems, including lack of a consent for the amputation of a leg. Finally, verbal consent was obtained from the patient's daughter. However, the doctor had obtained consent for amputation of the wrong leg! Also, the chest x-ray and EKG (electrocardiogram) were outdated, pre-operative urine had not been sent to the lab, and the anesthesiologist had not seen the patient. After explaining to the surgeon the lack of informed patient consent for anesthesia (which must be obtained by the anesthesiologist), the surgeon stated that the patient would have local anesthesia, and therefore did not need this legal form completed. Local anesthesia for an amputation? Not only is this type of situation frustrating and frightening, but there is no time built into the shift for handling these problems. Once these arise, the nurse usually loses her break time, and may very well work through eight or nine hours straight. It is no wonder that nurses burn out after being subjected to common situations such as this.

There are also emotional stresses which draw tremendously on the nurse's energy. A friend of mine, a psychiatric liaison nurse — Ms. Smith — at a local hospital, recounted this story to me. She was asked by staff nurses on a surgical floor to see a patient (Mr. M.) whose wife had just passed away. The nurses were very upset because Mr. M.'s doctor had decided not to tell him that his wife had died. The nurses felt that Mr. M. had a right to be informed of his wife's death. Ms. Smith spoke to Mr. M.'s physician and finally convinced him to tell his patient the terrible news. However, he refused to allow Mr. M. to go to his wife's funeral. Again, the nurses and Ms. Smith felt the patient had a right to go, and Ms. Smith consulted with two other qualified physicians, who determined that the patient was stable enough to go the funeral. However, Mr. M.'s physician remained adamant in his decision.

Ms. Smith spoke to Mr. M. and told him of his physician's decision. Mr. M stated, "If I don't go to my wife's funeral, I'll die." Ms. Smith relayed this statement to the physician, who told Ms. Smith that she was interfering with the care of his patient and that he would not change his mind. On the day of the funeral, Ms. Smith learned that at noon, Mr. M. stood up, stated, "I should be at my wife's funeral," and dropped dead.

This story demonstrates the helplessness that nurses sometimes feel. Often, there is a conflict between the wisdom and judgment of two professionals. When those professionals are a nurse and a physician, it is the physician who almost always prevails. In this case, the frustration felt by the nurses was the result of their knowledge that Mr. M.'s rights were taken away from him and that their own professional judgment was ignored. In discussing patient's rights, Leah Curtain states, "Although laws can protect certain aspects of human rights, there is a vast area that laws cannot protect. For example, the law can restrain me from killing you, but it cannot require me to respect your humanity — to treat you with decency, kindness, or understanding" (Curtain, 1982, p. 80).

Nurses, as health professionals, are faced with ethical dilemmas, such as this one, on a regular basis. Situations such as this wear the nurse down, until finally she is depleted of her energy.

There are other seemingly less significant occurrences in the hospital which lead to the same result — anger and frustration. Lack of cooperation from ancillary personnel is very upsetting. While working one weekend in a local hospital, I was caring for a patient who needed a transfusion. His blood count had dropped dramatically from the previous day. The technician in the blood bank was upset that I needed this unit of blood on Saturday! He wanted to know the reason the patient had not been transfused during the week instead of the weekend.

To explain this was annoying, and also a waste of time that I did not have to spare. To discuss the chronically inadequate supply of linen seems ludicrous, yet when one sheet, towel and washcloth are allowed for each patient per day if the patients are incontinent, this becomes another source of frustration. In cases like this, we must split plastic bags and use them on the beds in an attempt to save the sheet underneath. This is hardly the "professional" care nurses want to deliver, yet, these are the conditions under which we must labor. These are examples of "no-win," impossible situations. Most nurses only ask that they have adequate staffing and supplies to give their patients the kind of care they require and deserve. Is this asking too much? Apparently it is.

We've discussed how emotionally and physically exhausting nursing can be. Let's take a look now at the dangerous and even life-threatening situations with which we are faced. How often have we been exposed to, but unaware of, patients with tuberculosis, active hepatitis or even AIDS? It is not uncommon to care for a patient for one or even two weeks and then find out that the patient has a contagious disease. This can happen easily since many patients are admitted to the hospital with indefinite diagnoses, and while the various diseases are being ruled out, often no special precautions are taken until a diagnosis is confirmed.

This demonstrates to me an absolute lack of respect and concern for the welfare of nurses on the part of physicians and hospitals. If a physician is even slightly suspicious that a patient may have a contagious disease, why not place the patient on precautions prophylactically? When I posed this question to various physicians, a common response was that nurses were being "overcautious" and "excessively concerned." Also, many physicians feel that their patient will be upset if he or she is placed on special precautions of any kind. I can appreciate the need to protect a patient from unwarranted embarrassment or fear, but there must be more concern for nurses, and any other healthcare personnel involved directly with the care of patients.

The following is a classic case in which the welfare of the nurses and other personnel was not considered. Recently, while working on a medical floor with a group of students, I assigned a very ill patient, Mr. J., to a student. Mr. J. had numerous bedsores that had a foul odor, indicating to me that he was badly infected. When the doctors were confronted with the question of placing the patient on some form of isolation so as to protect Mr. J. as well as his caretakers, the doctors felt it was not necessary. We took the initiative to send cultures on the patient's wounds which proved to be very infectious. We then notified the Infectious Disease Committee who reviewed the case and decided Mr. J. required contact isolation. Contact isolation means that Mr. J.'s caretakers must wear gloves and gowns when in contact with his wounds and linen, and the linen must be disposed of in a special manner so that it will be laundered properly. If we had not taken the initiative to send cultures on Mr. J., we would not have taken the proper precautions and could have easily contaminated ourselves. The physician showed no concern for the nurses in this case — a clear example of nurse abuse.

Some physicians are more obvious about their lack of concern for nurses. A friend of mine who is a registered nurse was working in a doctor's office. A patient previously diagnosed with AIDS came to the office. The doctor not only asked the nurse to draw blood from the patient, but also requested an in-house CBC (complete blood count) which would have required the nurse to open the blood tube to take a sample. This test greatly increased the nurse's chances of contaminating herself. Because she was aware of the risk and she questioned the necessity of the test, the nurse refused to draw the blood. The doctor, rather than drawing the blood himself, then decided the tests were not necessary. This situation brings up some interesting questions: 1) Was it really necessary to request bloodwork on this patient in the first place? Obviously it was not since the doctor changed his mind when it became his responsibility; 2) Does this situation demonstrate a complete lack of concern for the welfare of the nurse, by exposing her to contaminated blood when it was not necessary? Again, obviously it does, since the doctor would have drawn the blood if it was imperative, and, 3) How does this situation affect the nurse? Needless to say, the nurse was very angry and upset with the doctor. The rapport and mutual respect that may have existed prior to this incident were negatively effected.

Of course, I am not advocating refusal to care for patients with contagious diseases. I do believe, however, that nurses and associated healthcare workers should not be exposed to contaminated blood or other body fluids needlessly, and they should be warned so the proper precautions can be taken.

Another area of frustration for nurses is the attitude held by many physicians that nurses are there to follow their orders blindly. In 1909, Beates noted that the nurse should "never attempt to appear learned and of great importance ... she should be able and willing to render intelligent obedience to the instructions of the attending physician, and carry out his orders to the letter" (Ashley, 1976, p. 21). It is interesting to note that Beates made this statement in 1909, yet current attitudes towards nurses have not changed dramatically. However, I wish I knew how many lives were saved as a result of nurses' refusal to follow orders blindly. Any experienced nurse who has worked in a hospital in July (when the new interns arrive) knows what a fiasco this scenario is. These new doctors write orders without having any idea how to write one properly. They don't know appropriate dosages of medications, untoward effects or antagonistic effects to other medications. The problem is so obvious to seasoned nurses and so potentially dangerous that, in one hospital in which I was employed, head nurses and supervisors were asked not to take vacation in July.

Many physicians are not able to accept the fact that an experienced nurse can be a tremendous asset to his/her care of the patient. Some are offended when a nurse suggests a particular therapy or treatment for the patient. The nurse has to "tread lightly" and be very careful in the way in which she approaches the physician. She is in a subordinate position to him and must "play a game" to obtain the order she needs to give her patient better care. Psychiatrist Leonard Stein has described nurse-physician relationships in terms of "a doctor-nurse game" in which a nurse must appear to be passive. In this game, any suggestion a nurse makes to a doctor must be masked in such a way as to seem as if it were his idea, and a doctor may not openly seek advice from a nurse.

A study published in 1985 reports that the "doctor-nurse game" described by Stein nearly 20 years ago, is still being played. A resident interviewed for the study commented: "I have seen nurses, who really know a lot more than the intern, kind of gently guide him (the intern) into making the right decision ... They make some very good decisions and make some very helpful suggestions sometimes ... It is like trying to guide the ship without actually taking hold of the wheel. There are nurses who are good at that" (Prescott, 1985, p. 83).

A nurse in the same study stated:

"You have to be very careful whenever you talk to them (physicians) that you are not telling them what to do. You have to talk to them in such a way that you are asking their opinion and 'work in' what you want to say without being overbearing or threatening ... make them think that the idea is partially in their mind too."

Surprisingly enough, this is summed up by a physician who wrote:

"Nursing is a very demanding profession. To start with, nurses must learn everything a doctor learns, so that whenever a situation arises that might develop into a mistake on the part of the doctor if the nurse did what the doctor ordered instead of what he meant to do, the nurse can distinguish the latter from the former and prevent the mistake from occurring. Then nurses must learn how to use this knowledge so that neither the doctor nor the patient is aware they possess it, for, in the former instance, it might cause the patient to lose confidence in the doctor, and in the latter, it might cause the doctor to lose confidence in himself. Finally, if, despite a nurse's best efforts, things are not going well between doctor and patient, and the nurse can't patch it up, the nurse must take the blame. Nurses are very patient. They realize their reward will not be in this lifetime, for to receive even a fraction of the recognition they deserve would be to lessen the importance of the doctor. Nurses often believe in reincarnation" (Conger, 1988, p. 62).

One day while working on surgical intensive care, my patient's blood count had dropped to a dangerously low level. I drew a sample of blood from him and sent it to the lab so that two transfusions would be prepared. When the doctor came to the unit, I asked that he write the order for a transfusion. The doctor told me not to transfuse for the time being. My impression was that if I had approached him differently, that is, if I had informed him of the patient's blood count and asked him what he would like to do, he probably would have ordered the patient to be transfused. It seems that it is often necessary to "play the game" in order to get what we need, and this form of nurse abuse can be one of the most degrading, since we are not able to act like intelligent human beings who are educated and clinically experienced.

Some authors feel that "the current shortage of

nurses may be partly due to frustration brought about through the inability to practice nursing as professional clinicians and teachers, to be valued as important members of the healthcare team, and to be duly rewarded for the care and comfort they provide their patients" (Aiken, 1982, p. 141).

The following case study concerns a new graduate nurse who became involved, quite innocently, in several ethical issues while working an evening shift on a medical floor. Sad to say, it is not an unusual occurrence in healthcare today.

During the evening, Ann Marie checked on a patient, Mr. B., and noticed that he was pale, sweating, cold and clammy. When she took the patient's vital signs, she found that his blood pressure was 110/40 as compared to his normal blood pressure of 160/100. He did not have a fever, but his respirations were shallow and rapid. Ann Marie called the private physician and asked him to come and see Mr. B. The physician told her to continue to monitor Mr. B. and to call him an hour later. She did so and reported that her patient's blood pressure had dropped slightly to 104/40, and his breathing was still shallow and labored. Rather than come to the hospital, the physician again told Ann Marie to monitor his patient closely and to call him if there were any significant changes in his patient's condition. A half-hour later, Mr. B. went into cardiac arrest. He was revived and transferred to the intensive care unit. Ann Marie documented all that had transpired, including her communications with Mr. B.'s physician. Mr. B.'s family, as well as the physician, were notified of Mr. B.'s condition, and they all met at the hospital soon after. The physician made a statement to the family that "If only the nurse had called me sooner, all this could have been avoided". The family was understandably very upset and decided to complain to administration, believing that the nurse had been negligent in her care. Ann Marie was called to the nursing director's office and asked if she had noted any unusual changes in Mr. B., and if so, why she had not notified Mr. B.'s physician. She explained that she had noted the change in the patient's condition, and notified the physician not once, but twice, and had documented all of this in her nursing notes. The director checked the nursing notes and found the documentation accurately described Ann Marie's description of the evening. However, the family was still not satisfied, and they demanded a full investigation. During the investigation, the physician denied that he had been called by Ann Marie and also asserted that she had falsified the nursing notes to back up her own story. It seems unlikely that the physician was being honest since he did not report Ann Marie to administration for either negligent care of his patient or falsifying the records until the investigation was brought on by the family. The end result is that it was Ann Marie's word against the physician's (Curtain, 1982, p. 255).

This situation is a sad and frustrating one for a number of reasons. First, here was a new nurse who had been slapped in the face with "reality shock," the reality being that the nurse must decide which physicians she can trust, and which ones she cannot. Already in her young career, her relationship with physicians had been tainted. She had functioned extremely well in a critical situation, yet her ability, indeed her integrity, had been questioned.

Doubtless irreparable damage was done to the nurse involved. While she handled the situation both professionally and responsibly, she still had to defend herself. She had a very negative experience that is bound to stay with her for the rest of her nursing career.

This incident is not particularly unusual, in that nurses are often humiliated, harassed and "abused." It is no wonder that dedicated nurses leave their positions and even their careers. Although the exact outcome of this story is not known, it is highly unlikely that Ann Marie was able to redeem herself or her reputation. When there is a conflict between a nurse and a physician, the nurse usually loses.

Another negative effect of the physician's actions is the fear and distrust of hospital care instilled in the family. As Leah Curtain (1982, p. 264) states in her analysis of the situation, "Dishonest conduct among health professionals results in distrust and fear. It undermines the basis of patient-professional relationships, damages the credibility of healthcare institutions, and destroys interprofessional relationships."

A major responsibility of nurses which is not often discussed is that of patient advocate. The American Nurses Association Code for Nurses (1976) (Article Three) states, "The nurse must act to safeguard the client and the public when healthcare and safety are affected by the incompetent, unethical, or illegal practice of any person" (American Nurses Association's Code for Nurses with Interpretive Statements, 1976). Therefore, the nurse has a moral obligation and responsibility to the welfare of her patient. Does this not also imply that she has a legal responsibility to refuse to follow a doctor's order if she feels it is unsafe or unethical? Since nurses are legally licensed and are not unskilled laborers who are following orders blindly, I feel nurses must follow orders only if they feel the orders are safe and will not unduly harm the patient in any way. It is difficult to instill this concept in nursing students, basically because they still have the concept that doctors are god-like and make no mistakes. Having been a nurse for many years, I can say with authority that doctors are human and do make mistakes, though some might argue the point. In fact, they should be thankful that nurses are educated and always present, because we serve as a system of checks and balances which results in safer care for the patient.

While working in a local hospital, a new physician ordered a gram of Lidocaine to be given to his patient for cardiac arrhythmias — directly, as an intravenous bolus or loading dose. The nurse refused to give the dose, stating that this dose of lidocaine would kill the patient. The physician then realized that he needed only 1/20th of the original dose. In this case, the nurse had a legal responsibility to refuse to draw up this large dose, since her first priority is to act to safeguard the patient.

The conflict lies in the fact that nurses may suffer severe consequences, i.e., disciplinary action, or even job loss, for exercising their professional responsibility. Part of the problem is that there is very little relationship between the responsibility. Nurses are expected to give optimum and safe care with minimum staff and supplies. We have little to no authority, and yet lives are dependent upon us. A good example is a case concerning intensive care nurses in Toronto in 1987. One night, three nurses refused to accept a critically ill patient to the intensive care unit on the basis that they could not safely care for the patient. They notified the admitting physician and their supervisor. The hospital suspended the nurses for three days without pay, so the nurses took the case to court. The court ruled against them, saying that "nurses are to obey first, and grieve later." The judgment demonstrated to the nurses that they were seen only as employees by the court and the hospital, and that they "must do as they are told" (Wilson, 1987, p. 21). Most nurses would have difficulty with this judgment, since a primary nursing goal is to render the safest care possible. When nurses are not allowed to practice their profession according to established standards, it becomes impossible for some to remain in the profession.

Another complex subject, one which involves emotional, legal and ethical issues, concerns patients who are irreversibly dying. Part of the problem is that many hospitals do not have a clear-cut policy concerning patients who have no hope of surviving. The other part of the problem is the reluctance of physicians to write the order "Do Not Resuscitate" (DNR). Because of this ambivalence, nurses are often caught in the middle, between the patient's and/or family's wishes for no extraordinary measures to be taken, and the wishes of the physician to do everything possible for the patient.

Leah Curtain (1982, p. 300) says it well when she writes that, "As a rule, irreversibly dying patients should not be subjected to cardiopulmonary resuscitation. Pragmatically speaking, it achieves nothing. All that results is more agony for the dying and lasting scars for the living. It is a degrading and unnecessary interruption of a person's dying." While family and patients have their own feelings to contend with, nurses are actually caring for these patients. It is frustrating to care for patients who we know will not benefit from our care. They require a tremendous number of nursing hours, precious hours that could be spent with patients who could benefit from our care. This may sound cold and calculating, but the truth is that choices must constantly be made as to who will receive transplants, who will be allocated time on dialysis machines, etc.

If a clear-cut order is not written, or a decision is not made, the nurse is then placed in the position where she must resuscitate a patient who she may believe should be allowed to die without interference. Often the verbal decisions conflict with the written, leaving nurses in a precarious and uncomfortable position. The nurses sometimes make a decision to run a "Slow Code," meaning there is no urgency to rush to a patient's room who has experienced cardiac arrest, and an excessive amount of time elapses before cardio-pulmonary resuscitation is begun. In this way, nurses can officially say the patient was "coded," but they know and intend that the code will not be successful. This is not a legal course of action for nurses to take, and they can be held liable because of it. To avoid this situation, the decision whether or not to resuscitate must be discussed with the appropriate persons and agreed to by all appropriate parties prior to the event of death. I have been involved with many cardiac arrests where there was a doubt as to whether the patient should be resuscitated, and CPR was in progress while someone was attempting to contact the patient's physician.

The following is an excellent example of the lack of communication between two physicians, and the resulting chaos that affected the nurses caring for the same patient. A student nurse was assigned to a patient who was not to be resuscitated. The resident had spoken to the family and had written the order "Do Not Resuscitate." On checking the orders later that morning, I discovered that the private physician had drawn a line through the order, and written "Error" over it. The student rightfully believed that the family had changed their minds, and the patient was then to be resuscitated in the event of cardiac arrest. However, the private physician still did not want the patient to be resuscitated, as he indicated in the progress notes that only supportive measures were to be taken. Yet, he did not want the order written.

After removing the student from the case, and informing the head nurse of the dilemma, we hoped the patient would not experience a cardiac arrest while we were obtaining a proper order. Eventually the private physician rewrote the order not to resuscitate. If the patient had arrested, we would have had to perform CPR, knowing that this was against the wishes of the family. It is unfair and unethical that nurses are placed in these compromising positions.

Other heart-wrenching situations occur frequently — one of the most difficult to handle occurs when a patient is alert, and oriented, yet dying from a terminal disease. Mr. R. was a patient on a medical floor who was dying from lung cancer and was respirator-dependent. He was extremely uncomfortable and was literally drowning in his own fluids. He continually attempted to disconnect himself from the respirator so that he would die. The staff was forced to restrain his hands so that he was helpless and extremely frightened. He kept begging to be put out of his misery, but morally the staff could do nothing. I found myself avoiding his room and hoping that his death would come quickly. He finally did pass away, but the effect on the nursing staff was devastating. Situations such as this are the true "reality shock" for nurses. No one can prepare nursing students for this type of experience.

Recently, while working on a busy medical floor during the 3 p.m.-11 p.m. shift, I observed that the ratio of nurses to patients was inadequate. There were 38 beds on the floor and three registered nurses. The floor was divided into three districts or areas, with 12-14 patients per district. The charge nurse was counted as one of the three nurses, and therefore had an assignment of patients herself. Within the first three hours of the shift, four new admissions and two post-operative patients arrived on the floor. The charge nurse was overwhelmed with paperwork, so I offered to admit two of her patients. The first patient, Mr. L., was a man dying from lung cancer. His wife and son were present and were extremely upset. Mr. L. had arrived on the floor at 4 p.m. and had not been seen by a nurse until three hours later. I was embarrassed and humiliated because I could not excuse the delay. The patient should have been seen on arrival to the floor. However, the nurses were involved with other important functions that required immediate attention. This is a common experience for most nurses, and it leaves them with many mixed emotions — anger, frustration, helplessness and feelings of being undervalued.

Based on the degree of education acquired by nurses, as well as the ethical, moral and legal situations in which we are placed, it seems clear that nurses' salaries should be exceptional compared to other related professions. However, they are not, and many theorists feel there is a strong relationship between nurses' salaries and the shortage of nurses in hospitals. It seems that the nursing shortage is worse than ever, yet the following facts would contradict this statement:

(1) "Overall growth in hospitals has been declining for the past three decades. Since 1950, the ratio of hospital beds to population has dropped by more than one-third" (American Hospital Association. Hospital Statistics, 1980, U.S. Bureau of the Census).
(2) "Since 1950, general hospital occupancy rates have declined significantly."
(3) "The nation's output of nurses has doubled in the past three decades" (AHA, 1980).

"Given the decreased hospital occupancy rates and the increased number of nurses in the past three decades, why is there such a shortage of nurses in our hospitals? One explanation is related to wages of nurses. We've been looking at the many stressful situations in which nurses are placed, yet nurses' incomes are not comparable with those of other occupations predominantly filled by women in significantly less responsible and stressful jobs. In 1979, nurses' salaries were "on a par with the national average salaries of secretaries, even though the educational preparation is considerably greater for nurses. Teachers, female professionals and technical workers earned more than nurses in the current market" (Bullough, 1983, p. 28). On the other hand, when Medicare was introduced in 1966, nurses' salaries increased dramatically due to third-party insurers, and "hospital vacancy rates also dropped rather dramatically from over 23% in 1961 to 9% in 1971" (Bullough, 1983, p. 27). It seems obvious, then, that if nurses were paid relative to their worth, there would not be a critical shortage of nurses in the hospital.

When we look at all of the stresses affecting nurses, it is no wonder that so many burnout, especially since most of the stresses are unnecessary.

I believe a cycle has been started, in a sense, and it is a cycle that is going to be very difficult to break. The cycle began when nurses left the hospitals because of low salaries, poor working conditions, and lack of respect from administration and physicians. Hospitals now are unable to replace the nurses, and as the staffing problem continues to worsen, nurses will continue to leave as the tension becomes too great. Hospitals have been turning to "band-aid" measures, such as hiring agency and per diem nurses. Although many of these nurses are dedicated, they are floated to strange floors in strange hospitals, and expected to function well. Quality of care is bound to be affected in a negative way, and the regular staff nurses become even more discouraged.

In order to break the cycle, hospitals are compelled to make offers that nurses find difficult to refuse. Some hospitals offer full-time salary, medical benefits and pro-rated vacation time for those nurses who are willing to work every weekend for twelve hour shifts. The positions that were available under this staffing scheme filled quickly, and therefore adequate staffing was assured every weekend. Since the staffing was assured, nurses knew they would not be overloaded when arriving at work, and therefore the work was much more manageable. These nurses are satisfied with their work situation, and those with whom I spoke have no intention of leaving. Of course, there are still problems and complaints, but overall the nurses feel they are being adequately compensated for the frustration and stresses they must sometimes endure.

As previously mentioned in this chapter, there are many forms of **NURSE ABUSE**. Most nurses join the profession because of an innate desire to help people, and they gain a great deal of satisfaction from doing just that. But in order to function professionally and competently, nurses have basic needs that must also be met, including provisions for adequate supplies, a feasible ratio of nurses to patients, salaries that compensate for the level of care rendered and education expected, and respect from physicians and hospital administrators for our wealth and breadth of experience.

If physicians and hospitals would treat nurses with the respect they deserve as professionals, supply adequate staffing and pay decent salaries, many of the abuses that nurses experience would dissipate, and **NURSE ABUSE** would be resolved.

References

Aiken, Linda (ed). (1982). *Nursing in the 1980s-Crises, opportunities, challenges.* J.B. Lippincott Co. Philadelphia.

American Hospital Association. (1980). *Hospital statistics.* Chicago: American Hospital Association.

American nurses association's code for nurses with interpretive statements. (1976). American Nurses Association. Kansas City, Missouri.

Ashley, Joann. (1976). *Hospitals, paternalism, and the role of the nurse.* New York: Teacher's College, Columbia University Press.

Bullough, B., Bullough, V., & Soukup, M.C. (1983). *Nursing issues and nursing strategies for the 1980s.* Springer Publishing Co., New York.

Cherniss, C. (1987). Professional burnout in human service organizations. New York, Praeger, 1980, as quoted in *Nursing Times.* Aug. 12-18; *83* (32).

Conger, B. (1988). *Bag balm and duct tape: Tales of a Vermont doctor.* Little, Brown & Company.

Curtain, Leah & Flaherty, M.J. (1982). *Nursing ethics: Theories an pragmatics.* Brady Communications Co., Inc.

Firth, H., McIntee, J., McKeown, P., & Britton, P. (1986). "Burnout and professional depression: Related concepts." *Journal of Advanced Nursing.* Nov.; *11*(6).

Levenstein, Aaron. (1980). "The adversaries." *Supervisor Nurse*, Vol. II.

Prescott, P.A., & Bowen, S. (1985). "Physician-Nurse relationship." Annals of Internal Medicine, 103 (July 1985) 129 as quoted in *Ethics in Nursing*.

U.S. Bureau of the Census. (1980) *Statistical abstract of the United States*. Washington D.C.: U.S. Bureau of the Census.

Wilson, Jane. (1987). "Why nurses leave nursing." *The Canadian Nurse*. March.

Chapter Eight

Nurse Work:
From The Eyes Of A Nurse Manager

What is it about being a nurse that leaves us disenchanted? What makes us dropout, quit, leave? Why do we feel the need to escape? The answer: abuse and stress. The relationship between abuse and stress is clear to nurses, or becoming clearer as we have entered the last decade of this century. The time has come for us to explain it to the non-nursing audience, which knows little of who we are or what we do — and to renounce anachronistic conceptions as relics of the past.

First, we must acknowledge the sources of **NURSE ABUSE**. Nurses in clinical practice know that these often encompass the entire working experience. It begins with the ever-present shortage of staff. Working on a busy unit and — recognizing the impossibility of having enough time or help to accomplish the tasks required — is another source. These circumstances do not promote an environment for a faithful adherence to the nursing process. It is unrealistic and unreasonable to expect that nurses tend to each patient, perform the routine care required — administer medications and treatments prescribed, meet deadlines for tests scheduled, and be available for each unscheduled crisis that occurs, not to mention the impossibility of administering the kind of excellent and educated care that nurses envision themselves delivering when they enter the profession. It becomes impossible for the staff nurse to update nursing care plans, perform audits and identify deficiencies in documentation, to name a few vital functions that would ensure excellence in nursing care. Patient teaching plans become burdensome and the likelihood of patient non-compliance ever more real. As our numbers decrease, the nurse/patient ratios increase. State and accrediting agencies have become more stringent in their documentation requirements, while pressure builds to levels that encourage an apathetic (or antagonistic) approach to paperwork.

The most frequently voiced complaints from professional nurses are a lack of staff and a lack of positive regard. The former is a constant reality in our present state of affairs. Increasingly, nurses are leaving the hospital environment for jobs in business, law, sales and the like. The most destructive influences, however, to the status of the clinical staff nurse are the other nursing positions in specialty services such as utilization review, quality assurance, patient advocacy and services such as IV teams, endoscopy specialists and non-invasive vascular studies. The clinical bedside nurse now witnesses a lack of parity based on workload, status and pay. If status and salary are indicators of one's significance, and in our society they are, then it becomes painfully clear that the closer one is to the bedside, the more insignificant her importance. An example: In one agency, positions were posted for X number of utilization review RNs requiring three years of clinical medical/surgical experience. More than 50 percent of the head nurses applied for these positions. Those who were selected were given the status of assistant supervisor, higher pay rates and a considerably lighter work load.

Who could question their choice? There is little advantage, indeed little incentive, to remain in a head nurse position, and be required to deal with a demanding public, be responsible to arrogant physicians, be held accountable for transcription and nursing errors, and be required to follow and impose on your staff prescribed procedures of documentation. It isn't that utilization review is so stimulating and rewarding a job that it would inspire more than 50 percent of the accomplished professional first-line managers to choose this position over front line patient responsibilities. I believe these choices are an attempt to relieve their intolerable stress and anger. I fail to recall my education teaching me that reward would be found in assuring compliance with the DRG (diagnostic related groups) discharge deadline. Of course, I do recognize that administrative positions are necessary. However, it is vital that we be aware that extrinsic rewards such as status and salary. also be given to the care givers. The clinical nurse must be recognized as one of the chief protagonists in the hospital hierarchy and it is she/he who must be rewarded as well.

Let's look at our system of promotion. The higher a nurse rises in level of achievement, the further she gets from the bedside. Or, more accurately, the further one gets from the patient, the greater her position of authority. If this incongruity ceased to exist, nursing could realistically expect the greatest potential from the bedside nurse, creating the heightened self-esteem and pride which are now sorely lacking. There seems to be a bifurcation in our profession. Why not use our awareness and creativity to redesign future practices?

Consider the self-esteem of an individual who is targeted for abuse simply because she is *there.* For example, the anger that the family of a sick patient feels because they haven't received the answers they require from the physician very often is transferred to the first available representative of the healthcare team — the nurse. Examples of nurse abuse stem from the interactions of many other varied segments of our system as well. When an individual is the first-line person to respond to a patient call, many times she is the recipient of the client's stress. I recall a situation which involved a patient who was admitted for a routine surgical procedure. The unanticipated and dire events that followed created a prolonged hospital stay filled with critical medical events. The nursing staff received the anger generated by this patient's family in addition to extensive abuse generated in the form of accusations of nursing incompetence. Variations in procedures, such as turning this patient on an inflexible every-two-hour schedule, were not tolerated by the family. One such situation involved attempts at cardio-pulmonary resuscitation being instituted on another patient. Demands for turning were expected to preempt the CPR. This scene may seem unreasonable to our lay public but all too real to the nursing community. Those nurses who became saturated either quit or were transferred into other departments; those who stayed were criticized and challenged by both the family and the physician. Nurses became the scapegoats and prime targets for the tyrannical abuse of a family seeking revenge. Supervisors and patient representatives were routinely summoned for crisis events and conflicts between staff and family members, and although the staff cognitively understood the anger generated by grief-stricken families, applying reason did little to resolve these conflicts. The greatest emotional damage was experienced by the nurse at the bedside. Stress took its toll, and the conscientious individual began to question her role and career decision. Others simply escaped to other agencies, or from nursing altogether. This scenario, and the impact it had were irreparable.

Perhaps years of training in psychology can help us deal with these and other similar events, but that is not the situation as it exists today.

There is a real need to re-educate society to the role of the nurse. One method could be a statement of purpose which would read as follows:

To our patients and their families,

Our role as professional nurses spans a continuum through which we would assess your status of health and illness, diagnose and intervene with nursing treatment or referrals. We will be your teachers and serve as liaisons between you and the hospital community.

We are responsible to carry through the treatments that are ordered by your physician and, along with your physician, we have the knowledge and ability to identify the results of these treatments. This is done by observing you, knowing the expected effects of each treatment and carefully documenting these results. Your physician takes this information and adjusts treatment.

We will, in addition, keep you clean and safe while you are with us, which is an additional aspect of care that we have assumed. We will orchestrate this care by delegating it to others whenever we deem necessary. We will appreciate your criticism of this care, but cannot be held either legally or personally responsible for the behavior of others.

Please allow us to practice our profession as we have defined it.

(Signed) The Professional Nursing Staff

The recipients of **NURSE ABUSE** are not only the staff nurses. Managers receive their share from their own staffs, physicians, families and their superiors.

There is a sense of impotence associated with management. One can recognize the needs of the staff and be in a position of planning, but the manager is ultimately under the constraints of the bureaucracy. Our system of promotion is based on the belief that the manager possesses the clinical skills, educational preparation and interpersonal capabilities to best fulfill the requirements of the organization. How unjust and frustrating to the recipient to achieve this position and then be perceived by staff nurses as having crossed over into a separate and adversarial camp. How unjust and frustrating to recognize subtle signs by the bureaucracy that suggest endorsement of this separation.

Many feelings of being abused deal with anger towards the public — anger at patients, families, other nurses and top-line administrators. For instance, if I introduce myself as a manager, I am fearful that you will not perceive me as the recipient of abuse. But, as a manager, I can relate to abuse and its result on the same level as any nurse. I am an expert on abuse. As a graduate of a hospital-based nursing school, I have and continue to experience **NURSE ABUSE**. I feel abused when anger is directed at me because there are insufficient nursing personnel. My anger is directed at supervisors, those who assume temporary responsibility for a shift rather than 24-hour responsibility and accountability. They are quick to tell my limited staff to "do the best you can." I sense failure and anger when feelings of servitude are apparent in my staff, for example: family member to nurse, "I know it's time for your dinner but it's also time to turn my mother!" I am also angry when a nurse is publicly chastised by a physician, then privately offered an apology.

A primary responsibility of the nurse manager, a function that is intrinsic to this role, is the mentor relationship that encourages the professional growth of the staff nurse. Situations that arise requiring on-the-scene direction, such as delegation of tasks, involve assertiveness training. Appropriate assignments to all levels of hospital personnel, nurse attendants, laboratory employees, and even volunteers can allow the nurse to carry through nursing responsibilities and lessen the likelihood of doing everyone else's job. Too often a nurse is exposed to the anger of a physician when laboratory studies are not reported as requested. The nurse manager is in the best position to guide the nurses, having been on the receiving end of such anger many times. There are two ways to handle this scene. One, the nurse could instruct the physician to direct his anger toward the responsible department, namely the laboratory; or two, the nurse could suggest that the physician assist her efforts in getting the laboratory to recognize its responsibility to the physician's order and the nurse's request. The staff nurse must recognize that it is not her responsibility to explain why the laboratory hasn't completed or reported a requested study. Why do nurses accept this as part of their role? Could it be that not all nurses experience a mentor relationship with a manager? An actual complaint by a group of nurses involved a supervisor "passing through" a very busy medical unit. On this particular shift the staffing was inadequate while the patient census and acuity were high. Respirators were alarming, patients were calling and loved ones were waiting to get necessary answers to questions they raised. The supervisor's simplistic response to the crisis on this unit was to remark that the soiled linen was left uncovered. This criticism was later followed up by a phone call inquiring into the staff's compliance regarding the soiled linen. How can such leadership style foster collaborative efforts, let alone a mentor relationship?

Other frequently experienced situations relate to

inter-unit staff crises. The perpetual conflicts between emergency services, intensive care units, and medical/surgical general nursing units abound. Units accepting patients for transfers-in are at conflict with those which are transferring-out. Rather than recognizing the central problem, which is the inability to cope with the workload, the units strike out at each other. The reasons for dissension are usually attributed to superfluous or vaguely related causes and not to the underlying problem. One hears reports that "they just dumped the patient," "they didn't care that we were at dinner" or — the ultimate excuse — "they had the doctor call and make us take the admission before we could handle it." We must learn to resolve these differences, care for each other and identify the stressors of one group or individual. In fact, each of us is confronted with difficulties that are similar but also unique according to our individual position.

We are abused by families of patients whose expectations of individualized care are not synchronous with the abilities of limited numbers of staff members to comply with these expectations. Aggressive acts from family members directed at nurses fail to distinguish between the nurse as a caregiver and the nurse as an individual. Nurses are there to meet all the needs, and it is simply not our doing that there is limited help to meet these needs. Rather than supporting our efforts, families and patients become adversaries of the nursing staff. They relate experiences of nurses falling short of their expectations, generalizing their anger toward the group as though we were without individual characteristics. Nurses are perceived as being responsible for every facet of the hospital experience. One revelation came to me when I critically reviewed a "patient satisfaction questionnaire." Questions read as follows:

Did the nurse respond to your call promptly?

Was your bathroom clean?

Were your meals hot?

Did the nurse introduce herself/himself?

Here is the frank suggestion that cleanliness and hot meals are the responsibility of the nurse. There is a clear need for re-educating the public to the fact that nurses do not clean bathrooms nor are they responsible for the temperature of the meal. This questionnaire was finally changed but unfortunately long after it had been in existence. Many people were educated to this error. Much of the animosity that the nurse confronts with patients and families is a result of misrepresentations of this kind.

Our academic experiences teach us to be autonomous and to interact with the patient and his family in order to achieve mutually set goals. There is no more sobering awakening than the reality of our situation. In reality the patient census is high, the assignment does not allow for any deviation from the rapid pace at which the nurse must function in order to get the work done. A patient crisis, such as a cardiopulmonary arrest or a hypertensive crisis, a patient who fell, a trip to CAT scan or a thoracentesis can set the nurse back and destroy any semblance of a schedule. This is not conducive to patient teaching, patient interview and family collaboration. The anger of the nurse stems from the dichotomy between what nursing means to the nurse and what nursing actually is. Calls for help from the nursing staff to the supervisors are met with statements such as, *"Do the best you can!"* This is not an appropriate response to a conscientious nurse. Her gut response is anger and despair, and the conviction that supervisors don't realize that "the best

I can" requires support. "The best I can" is so good that it can serve as a public relations marketing campaign for the hospital; "the best I am" is a lot, but don't leave me with half the staff to accomplish the minimum, and then expect "the best I can" to come anywhere close to "the best I am."

Adversary relationships also exist between the physician and the nurse. Today more than ever before there exists a hostile environment between these groups. The threat of malpractice prevents physicians from acknowledging error, and creates the need to seek another victim to blame. The nurse stands in a very convenient position for this form of abuse. The physicians-in-training have much to lose by making poor judgments. Every day there is another situation in which a poor choice of treatment ordered by a physician is identified. Nurses routinely take verbal orders whether or not the institution condones this action. There are many crisis situations that demand this practice, and nurses do not, in general, hesitate to follow verbal orders. But how many of us have been burned? How convenient it is and how common for a doctor to deny a verbal order, leaving the nurse responsible. Can it be that so many nurses misunderstand verbal orders? One hospital unit established a policy forbidding verbal orders. It was interesting to see how the nurses in this agency reacted. Many extended their authority and disregarded the policy. Their platform was that they "were thinking of the patient's welfare." Ironically the nurse now sets herself up to be hurt by transcending rules that were made to protect her! The nurse-manager, trying to inspire adherence to the rules, is then the subject of hostility from one's staff.

Even under the most supportive of nursing administrations there remains the omnipotence of the medical regime. What other segment of our society sees the yearly growing pains of each new influx of interns as does the staff nurses at their own hospital? Certainly the greatest abuse directed at nurses is a result of the yearly conflict between the new physician and the nursing staff. Interns who were mediocre in their first year now serve as supervising residents. This chief-like attitude prevails as their residency continues. In order for the resident to command a patient situation, the nurse now becomes the vehicle through which he achieves power. Attending physicians also are not spared my criticism. The well-ingrained doctor/nurse "game" has become the best method for communication, and the only method the nurse can use to accomplish her goals for unit and patient management. Less resilient nurses find this subservience intolerable and seek areas of employment which distance them from the one-on-one "power game" interactions that dominate hospital work.

The administrative level of the nurse-manager does not allow for shielding her staff from the abuse of others. There are managers who do not share these feelings and who use their appointment to distance themselves from their staff, but these individuals are not included in my discussion because I, too, believe they should not be managers. Those who are true management material share a common philosophy: Having been there, we are finally in a position to improve the status of the nurse, not by distance but by collaborative efforts.

The reluctance to remain a nurse-manager develops soon after the "honeymoon" phase of promotion. Initially, the promotion is perceived as recognition of one's assets: the tangible rewards of achievement. Once out of the uniform and into attire that suggests "success," the manager becomes divided from the general group of nurses that comprise the nursing staff. Administrators now have a central person upon whom to focus accountability, while subordinates view this position as so removed from their own that camaraderie is simply not achievable. How often does the manager hear "when you were a nurse ..." from physicians who personally witnessed the expertise that led to her upward mobility? The stress that consumes us is the result of the dichotomy of being in a position to work for our fellow nurses, yet meeting the non-supportive, reluctant group of staff nurses who are the intended recipients of your efforts. This experience is shared by all levels of management, from the clinical supervisor to the vice president for nursing. When I was offered the opportunity to write about **NURSE ABUSE,** I recognized that this term would be centered on the recipient of the greatest injustices — namely, the staff nurse. I believe, however, that all nurses are abused. My sensitivity to this reality allows me to identify abuse that is directed to all levels of nursing. My platform is to heighten this awareness.

As a nurse-manager, the nurse is in a unique position. She possesses the knowledge to perform nursing functions with expertise, yet must delegate these to the staff nurse. She is in the best position, however, to be accountable to her superiors for the acts of those to whom she has delegated responsibility. She manages her staff with a style that allows them to grow and be autonomous, and she is hopeful that each member of the staff will react to any given situation with logic and knowledge. When one falls short of this, she directs her goals to teaching the staff how to respond in the future. When a staff nurse is in a position that is unfair, unjust or personally damaging, the nurse-manager is there to act as a buffer. If she does not, then she is left with a professional who has been emotionally traumatized and it will be difficult, if not impossible, to erase the psychological injury. An example of this is the experience of a new employee recently off orientation. She was assigned to her unit on the 3-to-11 shift. The preceptor program had been completed and a phase of independence had begun. One evening, a surgical resident and his entourage of medical students arrived on the unit to perform a thoracotomy and place a central venous line in a patient. In retrospect it is clear that his own incompetence was the basis for his behavior, but this was cleverly masked by his demanding and degrading remarks to the nurse. She was criticized, dictated to, and humiliated in front of this audience of observers. Her only "transgression" was that she lacked the expertise and superior technical skills to set up for a chest tube and central venous line, and the knowledge to guide the doctor's hand in such a way that allowed him to truly believe that he had performed the procedures himself. Her inexperience with a manometer gave credence in the eyes of others to her incompetence. It didn't occur to anyone at the scene that the resident shared this lack of knowledge. I was her manager but was not working evenings. By the time I could reach her she was professionally destroyed. Her resignation symbolized my failure to undo the damage that had been done. Reports to this resident's director criticizing his behavior evoked only grudging nods of awareness and no indication that the resident would be chastised.

The question I routinely ask is, "How is a resident of two years superior to a nurse of five years?" Where is the justice? I am angry and frustrated that the nurse didn't exercise her authority to interfere with this crass performance and to return the abuse she received with the kind of responses that would indicate her own awareness of his incompetence. At the same time, I know that she was alone at this scene and may have lacked the confidence to be openly proud of her own professionalism and cognizant of the resident's lack of knowledge. Nurses seem to require longevity in order to be perceived as experts while residents require nothing. Who are the "good nurses?" Doctors see this group as those who can start intravenous lines, pass Levine tubes and troubleshoot problems and events. The word "troubleshoot" can be translated to mean "fix it yourself before putting the doctor on the spot." In my mind, the experience of this newly hired nurse gives credence to the reality that nurses are not recipients of positive regard by physicians. Rather they are victims of hegemonic and misogynistic behaviors.

Nurse-managers who are not supportive or effective need not be tolerated by the nursing staff. A progressive nursing administrator will respect the opinions and needs of the individual groups inflicted with a poor leader. Title does not necessarily reap security. The reality is that managers are continually proving themselves — a necessity in order to justify one's existence, and earn the privilege to lead a staff of professionals. At this level, corrective actions range from encouraging attendance at and offering courses in management, to private disciplinary actions, with the ultimate potential being one of terminating an errant employee. The nursing staff remains the most essential group in the hospital setting. This reality must be recognized by nurses themselves in order for them to appreciate the strength of their relative position. All measures to improve their professional experiences must be explored and operationalized. Recognizing our importance will help us shed he cloak of servitude, and ultimately help us see ourselves as self-assured, competent individuals. A clinical nurse, confident in herself, sees no supervisor as threatening or challenging, but instead as an intermediary and, ideally, a mentor.

The stress and abuse that the nurse-manager is subjected to may eventually lead to her reluctance to manage. If she cannot come to terms with the problems intrinsic to the job her tolerance will be short lived. Efforts are made by the nurse-manager to convince the staff that while discipline must be maintained, they will be supported and defended as well. Although enlightened nurse managers possess the authority to end the unjust treatment of individual nurses, in certain circumstances we are unable to undo the more pervasive and insidious abuse that continues to exist. It is extremely difficult to help nurses who are reluctant to value themselves, to adopt a self-concept that refuses to permit treatment of a shabby or patronizing kind. I have seen patients throw their meal trays at nurses because the food was less than they expected. My recourse is to refuse to tolerate such treatment, and to help the patients redirect their anger toward the appropriate cause. An intimidated nurse routinely accepts this barrage of anger, leaves the room and calls the dietary department from the nurses station. This response reinforces the patients' inappropriate behavior.

Staff nurses see managers as removed and safe from pejorative treatment. We are not, however, immune from abuse, and we are not the enemy. Promotion becomes a difficult position from which to function. The manager becomes sandwiched between the staff and the bureaucracy, unable to change either. The sources of abuse directed at staff nurses may vary somewhat, but are comparable to those directed at managers. Each group is left questioning their career choices and experiencing disillusionment in their value systems.

The greatest paradox in nursing is reflected by the essence of nursing as we know it and the actual role of the nurse as it has evolved today. The stress that affects each practicing nurse is reaching unprecedented levels. We want nursing to be what it has professed itself to be throughout our educational careers, but we discover, upon graduation, the reality, saturated with frustrations. We are plagued with the work we have to do on one hand, and the care we wish the system would allow us to give. Our frustrations are negatively rewarded by **NURSE ABUSE**.

What is it that allows us to continue? Maybe it's

our fervent hope and conviction that nurses can, somehow, better than anyone else, effect change for the better in this multi-dimensional world of ours.

Chapter Nine

Solutions

"If it ain't broke, don't fix it!" is a catchy phrase designed for those things — relationships, careers, ideas,
machinery or gadgets — which clearly function well. Unfortunately, it is not applicable to the state of the nursing
profession which is now, at least figuratively, "broke."

For decades — if not from its inception — nursing
has been adversely affected by the kind of academic
preparation inadequate to meet the rigors of the workplace
setting. And in that setting — primarily the hospital, but
also the home environment — the nurse has found conditions which militate against her best efforts to deliver the
kind of consistent, high-quality care she envisioned when
she responded to what most nurses consider to be a lofty
calling: the opportunity and the ability to care for the sick,
to tend the infirm, to heal the wounded, and to impart
both her empathy and her knowledge to a population
sorely in need of both compassionate and informed care.
Even the nurse who enters nursing for pragmatic reasons
— i.e., job security, the ability to juggle domestic tasks
with a part-time career, good benefits, etc. — is a rare
species, for she knows that these advantages will be
earned caring for those members of society who, through

accident or illness, have been deprived of their normally productive capacities — if not permanently, then at least temporarily.

She knows that she will be present and that her presence will be critical when there is pain, when there is blood, when there is trauma, when there is anguish, when there is fear and doubt, anxiety and depression, birth and death. And she knows that her presence will not be passive, that it will depend upon the highest level of knowledge, of skill, of judgment, of intuition and of alertness.

Yet, in spite of both the academic and clinical preparation she has had; in spite of the years of seniority she might have accumulated; in spite of her involvement in professional organizations; in spite of the additional degrees she may have earned; in spite of the ways in which her own interventions or diagnoses may have saved people's lives, in spite of her most impassioned efforts to change "the system" in which she works — the nurse finds herself entrapped, sometimes literally, in a job situation in which Nurse Abuse abounds. She is devalued, patronized, harassed, and, as a "bonus," underpaid.

As if this were not bad enough, the nurse of the 1990s finds that her situation has gotten worse. The need for higher wages, intolerance of poor staffing, thwarted efforts at organizing — all have brought about a defection of the nation's nursing population and a drastic reduction in the number of registered nurses in the nation's hospitals. In response, hospital administrations responded by revealing, for all the world to see, the depth of their contempt for the nurses who, before their dissatisfaction impelled them to leave, had been the lifeblood of the institutions in which they worked. Recruiting nurses from other countries and doubling or tripling the workloads of those who remained on staff are only two of the strategies which hospital administrations have employed to demonstrate how dispensable the registered nurse population was to their institutions. While it is true that some hospitals, finding these alternatives-to-nursing-care strategies ineffective, started to increase salaries and advertise heretofore unknown (or, at best, rare) benefits (such as tuition reimbursement or affordable housing facilities), for many nurses these changes represent a policy that is "too little, too late". They have already begun to pursue the many other "carrots" offered now to women in our society.

When the crisis in nursing reared its head, the persistent and insidious sexism, that has characterized nurse-doctor relationships throughout history again manifested itself when doctors went one step further than hospital administrations and, in a July, 1988 American Medical Association convention, proposed a "new class of workers" to the healthcare system — the Registered Care Technician (RCT), which they rationalized would "draw in more male workers who otherwise wouldn't be attracted to nursing" (Dentzer, 1988).

In response to the "nursing crisis," many nursing schools have closed and others have cut back drastically on both their teaching staffs and on their programs. Desperately, they have instituted "nurse recruitment" days, seeking out the high school senior population to inform them of the benefits that would accrue to both themselves and society if they choose to enter the field of nursing.

However, the disaffected nurse — she who has abandoned the nursing career she once cherished and of which she was so proud — has found that her intelligence, her clinical and organizational skills, her capacity for hard work, her incisive judgment, her ability to relate and her indefatiguable energy, are more highly valued in the business world she has now turned to, in the law school she has now entered and, sometimes, in the academic setting she has now chosen. And, in the bank which she visits, she is now contemplating IRAs and CDs and not agonizing over overdrafts.

This nurse, having despaired of any viable solution to the many problems she encountered in her job, has forsaken nursing for what she perceives as greener, emotional, economic and professional pastures. Has she been right to leave nursing? Has she chosen the only reasonable path for someone wanting to preserve (or, more accurately, recover) her sense of self-esteem, make a better living or flex her intellectual muscles and her decision-making capacities? Is she correct when, as one nurse has stated it, "in nursing, things will never change!" Maybe — at least for herself — she is.

But, what of the nurse who remains in nursing? In the world of the future, will she, like the dinosaur, be recalled as a species which became extinct, its function hardly remembered and no longer relevant? In today's world, is she condemned to demonstrate the veracity of the doomsday conclusion that things will never change?

Are there solutions to the problems that currently beset nursing? Are there ways to end Nurse Abuse? The answer is a resounding "Yes!" And they are many.

ACADEMIA — PROBLEM #1

Nowhere has the current crisis in nursing been more palpable than in those areas of the country in which hospitals have been forced to deny admission to patients because of a dangerously low nurse-patient ratio. Nurses, who with greater and greater frequency are "burning out," are either providing compromised care or leaving the profession altogether. The dramatic decline in hospital nursing staffs, the closing of nursing schools and the bleak outlook for increased enrollment in the schools that exist — all are invariably attributed to inadequate salaries and benefits and to the widespread dissatisfaction of those nurses whose contribution to the nation's health is almost consistently devalued.

However, analysts of this healthcare crisis have not included a central issue, perhaps *the* central issue, that accounts for this phenomenon. Specifically, nursing schools have failed to address themselves to the crucial issues which affect the very modus operandi of the nursing profession. Although nurses, for the most part, work in institutional settings, the schools that prepare them for their jobs fail to include in their curricula the tools essential to cope with or survive the rigors nurses must endure on a functional level.

Nursing education, unlike the ancient studies of art, of, science of the humanities, is a relatively new addition to the formal education process. And its history, based on the fact that nursing has always been a "female profession" (up until the recent past), has had a rather unique evolution. That uniqueness is a function of the many issues that historically has been, particularly problematical to women — issues such as economic worth, sexism and power, to name but a few.

It must be remembered that the founders of modern nursing — Florence Nightingale, Dorothea Dix, Louisa Schuyler — were "refugees from the enforced leisure of Victorian ladyhood ... to them, nursing training emphasized character, not skills. The finished product, the Nightingale nurse, was simply the ideal lady, transplanted from home to hospital. To the doctor, she brought the wifely virtue of absolute obedience. To the patient, she brought the selfless devotion of a mother ..." (Ehrenreich, 1973, p. 36). The model of the Nightingale nurse persisted well into the beginning of the 20th century, insuring that nurses were underpaid and "educated" according to the needs of doctors, hospitals and patients — not themselves.

And yet nursing remained attractive to women and, with time, some key changes did occur in the academic preparation of women. In 1940 and through that decade, after an unprecedented number of nurses were mobilized for World War II, nursing curricula underwent a major change. Formerly dominated by a focus on biologic systems, the curriculum now introduced the study of psychosocial issues. Soon after, as a natural result of these models, emphasis on the interpersonal process emerged.

During the 1950s, nursing education embraced the "holistic" concept "in which the patient emerged as a logical focal point of the content presented in nursing schools" (Riehl, 1980, p. 10). While the philosophical and functional applications of this change are still being tested by nurses, it was a concept that inspired at least some nurses to deduce that if the individual is important and if I, too, am an individual, then I am important as well.

In the 1960s, several novel nursing approaches were introduced into the nurse's education: a redefinition of the nurse's role; the notion that a nurse was defined by her function; and a patient-oriented concept based upon human needs. However, in spite of these changes, society at large was still keeping the nurse in her traditionally devalued place. As late as 1969, 75 percent of community hospitals paid nurses less than $7,500 per year.

During the 1970s, the two-income family had become a common phenomenon, fueled by the women's movement and its emphasis on female autonomy, by spiraling inflation, by rising expectations and by increased consumerism.

By 1977, four million of America's health workers

were women. While male doctors (92%) were the very highest paid workers in America (in the healthcare system), nurses were among the lowest paid. Notwithstanding these demoralizing conditions, nursing education continued to make adaptations which demonstrated a clear commitment to the better-educated nurse. Nursing schools began teaching their students Martha Roger's model of man/environment/energy interactions, Peplau's model of personality development and interpersonal relations, Hodgman's model of preventative intervention and Neuman's model which identifies leadership, research, systems, teaching, nursing, communication, health continuum and life cycle in its conceptual framework (Riehl, 1980, p. 11).

Since the mid 1970s, there has been an increase in nurses seeking doctoral degrees, partly to meet the demands of the institutions in which they teach or administrate and partly to fulfil personal goals.

In 1966, there were only three doctoral programs in nursing in the United States. In 1985, there were 35. And yet, the American Nurses' Association showed only 0.15 percent of the 1.7 million licensed registered nurses in the U.S. had doctorates and fewer than 21 percent of these were in nursing. In addition, in 1980, of the 2,500 nurses with doctoral degrees both in nursing and in other disciplines, only 7 percent reported research as a major activity (Institute of Medicine, 1983) and so the federal government discontinued its financial support of the doctoral nurse scientist programs. Many nurses who have obtained doctorates report that they are not perceived as true colleagues or as experts in their working experience. The need to legitimize nursing and to prove its value seems to be a prevailing theme. And the obstacles of economic inequity and sexism (both overt and covert) continue to plague nursing even as we are closer to the 1990s (Brown,

1985).

And so it is clear that nursing education has striven for change. But, to my mind, it has not focused upon its most important element — the nurse herself — or on the very environments in which the nurse practices her art and her skills — the hospital or the home setting. In what seems to be their inability to effect what scientist/philosopher Thomas S. Kuhn has called a "paradigm shift," nursing educators have failed to factor into their educational policies a genuine appreciation of the individual nursing student, in all her complexity, and including her own valuable life experience. They have failed to include in their curricula those subjects which would allow the nurse's individuality to swim, not sink, in the bureaucratic setting.

Yes, it is true that early nursing was not, could not possibly have been able to predict or anticipate the global changes — in society, in economics, in feminist thought, in technology, in the law, in ethics, etc. — which have taken place over the past century, and most particularly over the past 30 years. But even modern educators seem to interpret suggestions for change as a repudiation of all that has gone before. Is Kuhn correct when he states that "lifelong resistance, particularly from those whose productive careers have committed them to an older tradition ..." (Kuhn, 1970, p. 151.) accounts for one kind of failure to embrace a new paradigm? It is certainly not too late in the evolution of nursing to include those subjects which have been glaringly — and to the detriment of nurses everywhere — absent from the modern curriculum. For instance, where are the courses in feminism that give nurses a historical perspective about the social, psychological and economic ways that sexism has affected female feelings — and subsequent actions — in the professional sphere? Since 97 percent of nurses are female, this omission is glaring.

Contrary to popular opinion, people who go into nursing are keenly aware of the many significant differences between nursing and medicine — and have consciously chosen to pursue the one and not the other. Nursing has always been characterized as a "woman's job" and those who have chosen this path exult in that description. To most nurses, that description defines a heightened capacity to be empathetic, to be nurturing, to be understanding, to give, to care, to tend and to make critical judgments based on a comprehensive perception of the whole person. And yet nowhere to be found, especially on the bachelor's degree level, are the kinds of courses that shed insight, impart knowledge or discuss coping strategies about the uniqueness of women's history and the sexist traps the modern workplace presents.

Nonexistent are the business courses that teach the inner workings of the bureaucracy and how to navigate its hazards. With the exception of a briefly introduced schematic, detailing administrative hierarchy (on which, not so incidentally, few, if any females, appear), there is no discussion that introduces nurses to the notion that it is they who might aspire to true administrative power. In true Machiavellian form, hospital administrators have perfected the "art" of giving some nurses the illusion of power which, by advancing their status, endowing them with new titles, and thus making them members of the administration, ensure that they will never again be true advocates of nursing concerns. By their failure to alert nurses to this ploy and to teach her to fight against it, nursing schools cast themselves as abettors. Absent is the course in finance or economics that would prepare the nurse administrator to control her own budget or the staff nurse to bargain for wage and price benefits with authority. Never raised is the issue of public relations or the use of advertising and marketing that could inspire the nurse to be her own best image-maker. Most disturbing is the fact that nurses are never taught that they will be entering a business environment; that hospitals are, for the most part, in the business of making money (or, at least, balancing the books) and that they run with the same or a similar structure to most other businesses. Yes, they are in the business of caring for people, a somewhat loftier motive than many other businesses. But the mistaken notion (reinforced by nursing schools that fail to illuminate their students as to its inaccuracy), is that, somehow, such a place is operated by people of unique, benevolent and even philanthropic instincts who will treat them with the respect they are due. In fact, hospitals are operated by businessmen whose prime motives are those that concern all businessmen — economic health and good public image.

Nowhere to be found in modern nursing schools is the law course that will teach nurses about their basic rights or how to redress grievances through legal channels. Much of the intimidation nurses suffer is a result of ignorance about the law — and how it pertains to their work (or life) situation. A good number of nurses have become lawyers and now represent other nurses to resolve their grievances. Are nursing students taught of their existence? Told how to reach them, should the need arise? Certainly not as a matter of policy.

It must also be remembered that nurses deal daily with the gravest medico-legal issues of our day. The care of AIDS patients, euthanasia, abortion, organ transplant, life-support systems, informed consent, patients' rights, the conflict (in some cases) between medicine and religion — all these issues and the myriad questions and conflicts they raise confront the registered nurse many times in her career, sometimes on a daily basis. And yet, in most nursing schools, there is not one required philosophy course until the doctoral level.

And it is a rare course that even mentions the power and efficacy of political action. Except for an occasional classroom "guest" who urges the student nurse to join a professional organization or to sign a petition, there is no mention of one of society's most dynamic means of effecting change — the political process.

To be sure, nurses are introduced to the lofty precepts that touch upon the subjects of feminism, business, law, philosophy, politics, etc., but, for the most part, this introduction is theoretical. When a random nursing student actually puts the theories into action, she is rarely supported either by her peers or the educators who have propounded them. Rather, she is considered somewhat of a rebellious curiosity, more valued as an amusing iconoclast than as a paradigm or an inspiration. This situation is all the more regrettable in light of the modern nurse's excellent preparedness in other areas. While she is ill-equipped to serve her own best needs, she is superbly equipped to serve the patients.

The registered nurse of the 1990s has, at minimum, an associate degree which includes a two-year, supervised clinical experience. Increasingly, she (or he) has either a bachelor's or master's degree education that includes studies in the social sciences, biochemistry, physics, statistics, physiology, biology and pharmacology, and also in the vital aspects of daily patient care. She must have a sophisticated knowledge of monitoring, suctioning, dialyzing and intravenous devices and routines, and also an in-depth knowledge of the great variety of modern medications, their actions and untoward reactions, and of intervention protocols.

And, because so many patients are now discharged from hospitals in serious condition, the modern home health nurse must embody an even greater degree of independent judgment, away from the aegis of the "protective" environment of the hospital. In addition, the modern nurse must also carry malpractice insurance which places culpability for patient care solely in her domain. Today, many nurses practice independently as psychotherapists, midwives, and pediatric and family practitioners. Others are university administrators and professors, community liaisons. The list goes on.

Several persuasive studies have shown that nurses who share power (i.e. decision making, nursing diagnoses, administrative input, control over their own budgets) have greater job longevity and satisfaction than those who are employed and exploited by places that do not demonstrate a similar respect. While wages are, indeed, a major issue, it is clearly not the arch-criterion by which nurses judge the value of their jobs. Even when salaries increase, grievances persist. Certainly, the pernicious sexist hang-over which characterizes administrative intransigence accounts for some of the dissatisfaction. However, many of nursing's problems are the result of the contradictory and self-abnegating lessons which have been foisted upon generations of nursing students: "Yes, you're valuable, but don't tell anyone — you might alienate them." "Yes you deserve more pay, but don't demand it — you might lose your job." "Yes, you have a superior body of knowledge and legal accountability, but don't make waves — you're dispensable." These destructive "messages" in conjunction with a uniformly inadequate curriculum conspire to put all nurses at a disadvantage" (Swirsky, 1988).

ACADEMIA — SOLUTION #1

Nurses are more than the sum of their parts —

their choice of career, their clinical function, their specialty area, even their uniforms. Nursing education must introduce this concept to nurses on more than a didactic level. For instance, it has always struck me as odd and limited that, at the beginning of each semester, when and if nurses are asked to introduce themselves to their classmates, they are never expected (or encouraged) to include anything about themselves outside of their nursing experience. In over 17 years of sitting in nursing classrooms, I have rarely heard anything in these introductions other than, as Sergeant Friday would say, "the facts, ma'am." "My name is Jane Doe," a typical introduction would begin. "I work at Queens General Hospital in the ER. Before that, I worked at Stony Brook Hospital in the ICU. Someday, I'd like to go into administration." What, I wonder, does this person do in her leisure time? What outside interests does she have? What kind of music does she like? Is she involved in any volunteer activities? Is she political? Artistic? Mechanical? A skydiver? Does she have children? If so, how many — four? Nine? If these and other facets of her life were elicited, if she were given the impression that they really do define her more fully, then perhaps she would be encouraged to implement the qualities she brings to other pursuits to the pursuit of nursing.

For example: she might bring the courage of skydiving to negotiations with the administration; the love of music to her patient's bedside; the volunteer impulse to that "extra" gesture; the skill at juggling domesticity with academia and nursing to administrative tasks. Too often, concepts taught in the classroom are learned but not incorporated. When they are personalized, they become more "real," and thus more applicable. If nursing faculties made it their business to learn more of the vital living experiences of the nursing student, they would affirm to the student nurse that her personal frame of reference and the lessons she has learned have value — the kind of value that she might take into the clinical setting. In modern nursing classrooms, this facet of the educational experience is certainly not the norm.

In addition, nursing curricula must be revolutionized to include subjects (again, such as feminism, business, ethics, etc.) which have direct relevance to the nursing experience. But where, one may ask, will "the experts" in fields such as business, law, feminist thought, philosophy, politics come from? Simply, from other institutions or from the public sector where they exist. Why must nursing schools, unlike other centers of higher learning, rely exclusively on their existing faculty or draw only from their own discipline — or from an occasional lecturer from the outside world? There is a vast wealth of resource people available to impart information based on their areas of expertise. Nursing schools must find these people and utilize them wisely if the nurse of the future is to be equipped, in all areas, for the job she will perform.

But what of the courses that already exist? In the case of many — get rid of them. Nowhere can more "dead wood" be found than in current nursing curricula. Nursing schools must stop teaching small group process, problem-solving techniques, assertiveness training, and all the other narcotizing courses that teach nurses more how to "behave" in the system than how to prevail in it.

Also, there must be a better system of evaluating faculty. There is not a nurse who cannot recount a tale of at least one teacher who was ignorant, uninformed, punitive, competitive with her students, intolerant, lazy or terminally boring. And yet, in spite of mandatory evaluations at the end of each semester, that same teacher continues to contaminate the classroom with her inferior teaching or her mean-spiritedness and to waste the valuable time of the nursing students, many of whom hold full-time jobs and/or raise families. What does the administration do with these evaluations? Do its members visit the classroom, on occasion, to evaluate for themselves the truthfulness of such negative reports? Do they suggest relevant courses (in human relations, for instance) or recommend psychotherapy to the teacher so evaluated, the better for her to alter her behavior? Do they review the tenure system to find ways to relieve such a teacher from her classroom tyranny? Clearly, these strategies are infrequently, if ever, employed — for this kind of teacher, like death and taxes, is always there, a given in human existence. But need they be? I think not. Here, too, action is imperative if the seeds of nurse abuse are to be eradicated.

In terms of required texts, it is important to mention that many "authoritative" sources continue to employ gender-biased language. When a nurse reads that "man believes" ("thinks," "feels," "postulates," etc.) or any of the other statements which imply that action and thought almost unilaterally derive from the male of the species, there is the very real feeling that what she has read precludes not only 100 percent of most nursing classes, but 97 percent of the nursing profession as well. While some modern texts are written or edited with a sensitivity to the universality of most experiences, most continue to be riddled with statements which both assert and imply the primacy of male thought and experience. The subtle yet powerful message which this kind of language conveys — and which suffuses most writing — cannot be calculated in terms of the demoralizing effects it has on the women whom it clearly does not address. It behooves nursing instructors to be sensitive to this issue and to seek out those texts which do not reflect such flagrant and destructive gender bias.

POLITICS — PROBLEM #2

As nursing has evolved over the centuries, and particularly since the early 1900s in America, it has gone from a profession which was characterized by servility, self-abnegation, obedience, passivity and dependence to one which has been developing into an active, assertive, self-defining and independent force to be reckoned with. And yet, even now, in the 1990s, after literally decades of social ferment and revolutions both economic and sexual, nurses do not wield the "clout" which other, more aggressive constituencies have found in our political system.

Political action is not new to nursing. Early nurses such as Lillian Wald, Lavinia Dock et al., were politically involved, and nurses since that time have attempted — and with some measure of success — to affect important changes through political action.

With the advent of Nurses for Political Action in 1971 and the eventual absorption of that group into the ANA's N-CAP (Nurses Coalition for Political Action), nurses began to have some power, however limited, in public policies which affected their professional lives. And, the Nurse Training Act of 1971, among others, took on the responsibility for enforcing provisions of laws prohibiting sex discrimination.

Even before that, the feminist revolution of the 1960s brought about several important changes. The institution of NOW (National Organization for Women) spearheaded long-overdue legislative change. Using Title VII of the 1964 Civil Rights Act which prohibited economic discrimination on the basis of sex, NOW and other organizations worked effectively to tear down ancient barriers which excluded women from equal access to good jobs.

Over the last decade, there has been a significant increase in independent nurse practitioners, many of whom have become involved in the political process, the better to propose, support or fight the legislation necessary for them to survive and flourish independently. There has been a spate of lawsuits which have focused on academic grievances and workplace inequities. And there has been growing numbers of nurses (including students) who have plunged into the political process.

Organizations have proliferated. Rules and regulations have been formulated. And, indeed, some important legislation has been passed. Greater number of nurses are now participating in the political process — be it as members of professional organizations, "grass roots" activists, lobbyists or organizers. If one is looking for examples of greater participation, it can be found. However, considering that there are almost 2 million registered nurses in this country, the vast potential of nursing as a political "force" is still greatly underrepresented in the political life of our nation.

It may be that the kinds of people which nursing attracts are, by nature, apolitical — more attuned to giving than to taking, more comfortable with meeting the needs of others than in expecting or demanding that their own needs be met. Perhaps it is the perception of a personal powerlessness that prevents many nurses from seeking solutions to their problems in an arena in which the assertion of power is a given.

People who are politically active almost consistently entertain the notion that they, personally, can do something to make a difference. They believe that through their vote, their participation, their involvement, they can effect (and affect) change at the very source of the problems facing them. Whether they are issues as sweeping as war and peace, crime, health reforms or day care, or such issues as hiring and firing policies or equity in pay — all are larger than the individual who faces them on a daily basis. It is only through political activity that these issues can be addressed in any meaningful way in our society, precisely because it is only through our legislators (and the legislation they either do or do not enact) that both our needs and desires can be met.

Although there have always been notable examples of nurses who have appreciated the power of political action, involved in such action themselves, by and large nurses have been apolitical. Why is it that the clear cause-and-effect lessons that political life demonstrates have been so long in reaching nursing consciousness?

For many years, the ranks of nurses came from a population of women who, while aspiring to some sense of identity outside of the home, were attracted to work largely perceived as extra-domestic — nurturing, care-taking, subordinate to authority. Even in the 1970s, the choice of nursing as a career did not include the search for an education which went beyond the bounds of "training." With the reevaluation of nursing curricula and the subsequent decision to standardize entry-level requirements to include a baccalaureate degree, a "new" kind of nurse was envisioned — one whose education would include at least a dabbling in the humanities, the social sciences, the historical "trends and issues" which preceded decades (in fact, centuries) before.

This alteration in philosophy and direction coincided with the feminist revolution and the sweeping changes in the structure of our society. As female-male relationships underwent a metamorphosis, as more than 50 percent of women entered the work force, as medical technology exploded in a proliferation of new treatments, machines, expectations and responsibilities, the decision of nurses to place themselves in the context of modern society came not one minute too soon.

But, before then, the education of nurses was tailor-made to fulfill the roles which they were expected to execute as auxiliary healthcare providers and passive recipients of orders and directives. It is no wonder that, up until the last decade, most nurses (again, with notable exceptions) had a limited awareness of the power of political action.

And so, one reason — perhaps the major reason — why nurses' participation in political life had been so inadequate until the past several years is because they were simply never taught that there were political strategies, both inside and outside of the hospital, by which grievances could be effectively addressed. Even today, the sluggish wheels of bureaucracy continue to reinforce to nurses the message that their efforts at change are, more often than not, an exercise in futility.

The hospital situation is a good example of the kind of discouragement which nurses face almost daily. In most institutions, nurses are taught to address their grievances to the nursing supervisor or head nurse. In the Machiavellian way mentioned before, hospital administrations have figured out exactly how not to share power. They have done this by making supervisors and head nurses part of administration. They have made the rewards for these positions irresistibly attractive to nurses — both economically and in terms of status — and they have made the consequences (if the now-elevated nurse should depart from the administrative "party line") most unattractive, even threatening. The result is that the staff nurse whose goal it is to redress a grievance or to bring about a change of policy must address a superior whose loyalty is, at best, divided and, at worst, adversarial. In a too-typical scenario, the nurse who needs an advocate or who wants to resolve a problematic issue finds herself on the receiving end of delaying tactics or embroiled in endless meetings in which the net result is a minimum of satisfaction and a maximum of frustration. A "can't-fight-city-hall" mentality develops as the nurse's anger and frustration are met with the proverbial "lip service," patronizing inattention, or the kind of irritation usually reserved for buzzing gnats. If she does not "identify with her oppressor," get depressed or increase her dosage of Maalox, then she either drops out of nursing or else she goes on for an advanced degree where the whole process is elevated, not changed, to a "higher" level. Conditioned to believe that they are essentially powerless, it is no wonder that more nurses are not attracted to political action. After these kinds of experiences, it is fruitless to talk to the nurse of the "power" which political action can yield. Power feels good. But like any other asset, it only feels good to the person who recognizes that it exists. It is as meaningless to tell a beautiful girl who thinks of herself as ugly to get a modeling job as it is to tell a nurse who feels powerless to exercise her power.

Nursing perpetuates this sense of powerlessness by asking of itself the wrong questions. While we debate whether nursing is, indeed, a profession, are we not straining at a flea and swallowing an elephant? If we do not enjoy the privileges of professionalism, is the debate relevant? In the same sense, is it important for nursing to ask what job titles afford the most prestige, if all job titles are essentially powerless in the hospital hierarchy? And, yet again, is it crucial for nursing educators to ask for increased science courses in their curricula if its nurses are not considered equal partners in the prevailing healthcare system and, therefore, are not called upon to share or practice what they've learned? In the clinical experience of most nurses, the unique knowledge they have is curtailed by a complex system of medical, legal and sociological restraints. While a nurses' observation, for instance, may denote that a particular regime is called for, that a combination of medications is having an untoward effect, that a particular therapy is indicated, she cannot implement action or act on her knowledge independently. She is impelled to pass along her observation to a variety of medical specialists who then act on her advice and observations to the benefit of the patient. Of course, it is they who receive the positive feedback (if not downright adulation) that the good treatment has inspired. The nurse's practice is severely compromised. She is left with the rules, while others take the action. Again, how can the nurse perceive herself as powerful if even the real power she has is appropriated from her?

Is this bleak picture a blueprint for the future of nursing? Too many hopeful possibilities exist to draw that conclusion.

POLITICS — SOLUTION #2

In nursing schools and in the workplace, the subject of politics must be made a central issue, introduced as the vehicle through which major changes can be made. Once the structure and function of government are understood, the issues must be articulated. Are independent nurse practitioners allowed third-party payment privileges in my state? Where is the resistance — from the medical community? The insurance companies? Are sexist clothing codes being sanctioned in my place of work? Are non-professionals or paraprofessionals allowed to perform nursing functions — in spite of their non-licensure? Are hospitals violating union agreements with impunity? The list of political issues, as they affect nursing, goes on. In order to address them politically, they must first be known.

Again, both schools and the nursing administrations in hospitals could offer credits or CEUs for the nurse who mobilizes a constituency — in politics, there is strength in numbers. Nurses with political experience could teach mini-workshops to demonstrate the actual "how-to" of political action — letter-writing campaigns, lobbying, phone calls and visits to local legislators, media advertising, fund-raising. And, most important, nurses must make their needs — and especially their voting power — known to local, state and national politicians. It is truly amazing how attentive politicians are to those blocs which express their most fervent desires in the voting booth.

In a political action organization to which I belong, candidates are interviewed personally (at the homes of members of the organization) and queried as to where they stand on the issues most central to the organization's philosophy. In our view, there are right answers and wrong answers to our questions, and we take the opportunity to educate the politicians in the event that their answers are either misguided or antagonistic. In just a few short years, we have found the politicians using us as resource people and utilizing our endorsements in their advertising campaigns. It matters to them that we vote. And, because of our interviewing and endorsement policy, letter-writing and phone call activity, and the numbers of people who are sympathetic to our philosophy (all of whom also vote), we find their responsiveness increasing significantly each year.

The political process is available to all people. But, like all processes, it needs to be learned, to be practiced, and to be implemented. When nursing enters the political mainstream and becomes a force whose voice (vis-a-vis votes) demands recognition, the issues which can only be dealt with only on a legislative level will earn the responsiveness they deserve. And, when the principles of political action are applied in the work setting, additional progress will be made.

PROBLEM #3 — FEMINISM

Throughout history, women have worked in outside-the-home jobs.

In this country, even before they pursued the "traditional" jobs of teacher, nurse and secretary, women worked in "mom-and-pop" enterprises, at home in "cottage industry" pursuits, in sweat shops, in mills and in the fields. In 1900, almost all women workers served as domestics, farm laborers, unskilled factory operatives or teachers. And yet, by 1920, in spite of the suffrage movement, traditional attitudes remained fixed, jobs remained segregated according to gender, and women's jobs were defined as "woman's work."

The economic and social history of women in this country is also the history of nurses. However, because nurses were among the first to enter the labor force, their grievances are particularly galling. Throughout the decades of the 20th century, nurses have been heiresses to all of the biases, wage discrimination, sexist thinking and acting that have plagued the larger population of women as well.

Within four years from the start of World War II, more than 6 million women entered the job market in response to an unprecedented demand for new workers and new production. Nurses were among the most populous of the new work force. At that time, the government, in support of the need for female workers to compensate for the men away at war, allocated $6 million dollars for war nursery schools. When the war was over, many women chose to remain in the work force, so beginning our current system of the two-wage family.

For one thing, many of the women who then chose work outside of the home did so only when their children were of school age. In addition, because our society was less mobile, working women could frequently count on family members or friendly and trusted neighbors to care for their children. Also, the one-parent family, a by-product of the "divorce mania" about to sweep the country, was then a relatively rare phenomenon. It would not be long before divorced women would enter the work force out of the sheer necessity to insure that both they and their children would survive.

During the 1950s, twice as many women were on the job as in 1940. However, even as more women were pursuing professions once held to be the exclusive domain of men, society at large was keeping woman in her traditionally devalued place. The disparity in pay scales remained wide and few opportunities for advancement remained enduring obstacles.

And then, in 1960, came The Pill, the feminist movement and the sexual revolution. With the advent of the birth control pill, women forsook early marriage in order to explore the increasing variety of opportunities which loomed on the horizon of a changing society. The feminist movement fueled these efforts, reminding women that, by controlling their own biological destinies, they could now concentrate on other facets of their development. As the feminist movement took hold, "traditional" roles were called into question on all fronts — economic as well as domestic.

Many women now deferred marriage and motherhood in pursuit of a career. Some found themselves in satisfying careers, many of which demanded great responsibility and an obeisance to "the rules of the game," namely no children. Those who chose to have children found that they were living in the only civilized industrial nation in the world which had no national system of parental leave. With increasing economic independence, women who had once languished in bad marriages (or in non-marital relationships), had the ability to leave them. As the divorce rate rose (to one out of two marriages), so did the standard of living. Women who were single parents found themselves sole breadwinners. Married women, many out of economic necessity and others out of the desire to attain satisfying careers, became part of family complexes in which two salaries were required to fulfill a viable standard of living. Many who were divorced, found themselves on the receiving end of flouted child-support payments and with no viable means of maintaining their families other than joining the work force. Others, with husbands and children, found that one salary was inadequate to meet a growing family's needs. And still others chose to combine career and family, feeling that they could do justice to both.

During the 1970s, the two income family had become a common phenomenon, encouraged by the women's movement and its emphasis on autonomy, by spiraling inflation, by rising expectations and by increased consumerism. Yet through all this change, some things remained the same. The vast majority of women continued to work in sex-segregated occupations, concentrating in service industries, female clerical jobs, government positions, manufacturing, teaching and nursing. Also, women continued to be denied access to decision-making and executive positions or to have job-related necessities (such as maternity leave or day care) addressed with any degree of support or seriousness.

Now, in the 1990s, with increasing numbers of

women entering the work force — and becoming mothers — many of the inequities of the prevailing system still have not been effectively addressed. In the vital areas of pay equity and advancement opportunities, progress has been sluggish. And in the area of day care, problems of inadequate legislation, of meager funding, of poor regulation, of underpaid staff workers abound. Concerns as to the psychological effects of day care on children less than one year of age, on toddlers and older children and on the mothers who must juggle parental and economic responsibilities — all are in question.

Today, according to Edward Zigler, director of Yale University's Bush Center in Child Development and Social Policy, three-quarters of the nation's working women have school-age children; half have infants less than a year old. And yet, in spite of the radical changes which our society has undergone in the past three decades, all the issues which plagued women in the 1960s are alive and well in the now, with some of them, such as the intransigence of male "role" behavior having become more exaggerated and infuriating with time.

A major study, undertaken by the Congressional Budget Office, found that American families are better off than they were in 1970 but that those families with the lowest incomes, including single mothers with children, "became worse off during the period" from 1970 through 1986. Overall, the median adjusted income of families in 1986 attained the highest level on record; for families with children it rose 14 percent, but for single mothers with children, it rose just 2 percent. This last, bleak statistic, compounded by the Census Bureau's 1987 report that the average weekly wage of women workers was 70 percent of what men earned (in 1986), highlights the continuing contempt and devaluation of women in our society. Since nearly one American youngster in four (14.8 million children) lives with just one parent (89 percent with the mother), it is clear that the demands, needs and expectations of women — even when it comes to the care of their children — is similarly devalued.

Presently, job-protected, paid maternity leaves — most of them very brief — are available to fewer than 40 percent of employed mothers.

Groups such as the National Federation of Independent Businesses and the National Association of Manufacturers oppose the concept of parental leave, citing issues of cost and the threat to employee relationships. Given this information, it is not surprising that, in a report in May, 1988, the Census Bureau said that the inability to find a babysitter disrupted the jobs of about 450,000 women nationally each month.

According to economist Sylvia Ann Hewlett (1986, p. 97), "women are joining the European work force at much the same rate and for much the same reasons as in America. But there is one major difference. In Europe, working women are supported by an elaborate (and in most cases expanding) family support system which is a major factor behind their improved earning power. It is no coincidence that the country with the most developed benefits and services for working women — Sweden — is also the country with the smallest wage gap, while the country with the least developed benefits and services — the United States — is also the country with one of the largest wage gaps."

In spite of some grand protestations to the contrary, it appears from looking at the actual state of women's employment in our country, that the oldest and most destructive stereotypes about women and about the task of caring for children have not significantly improved. "Woman's work" has, for the most part, been considered primarily that of childbearer and child-rearer. Historically devalued, it has also been perceived by many women (at least those who have identified with their detractors' definition of worth) as a job somehow intrinsically less valuable than that of wage earner. Now, as more and more women pursue that male-defined characterization of success — the salary — they find that society is wildly out of sync with their most cherished fantasies about how both they and their children will be perceived. Rather than the heightened esteem they have been led to believe accrues to those who "earn a buck," women are finding that neither they nor their job status have affected, to any satisfactory degree, the system — of employers, legislators, pay scales, benefits, etc. — which reflects their hard-fought-for but not-yet-won full entry into society. When it comes to the issue that is paramount to their concerns — the welfare of their children — the full impact of this lack of esteem looms largest.

Nurses know these grim facts as well as, if not better than, the rest of the female working force in America. Is this issue too big for the nurses of our country to handle? Decidedly not.

FEMINISM — SOLUTION #3

Roots! Women must learn from whence they came in order to know in which direction they want to go and in order to appreciate the formidable historical, social, cultural and psychological obstacles which stand in their way. In the case of nurses, it is incumbent upon every nursing school to incorporate into its curriculum courses on feminism — feminist thought, philosophy, history. It is important for the nurse to understand how being a woman has affected every facet of her life — from the Bible to the ERA, from the first flicker of the Nightingale lamp to the last check she made out for malpractice insurance.

If Carol Gilligan (1982, p. 160) is correct (and I believe she is) when she says that "... the female comes to know herself as she is known, through her relationships with others," then it is clear that when the nurse is devalued (abused) in the workplace and in society in general, she comes to devalue herself. Conversely, if strategies were devised to lead the nurse to reevaluate herself in positive terms, her image of herself would be immeasurably enhanced, both personally and professionally.

On a personal level, nurses can form "consciousness raising" groups, in which experiences are exchanged, common problems are discussed, solutions and strategies are formulated and support is shared.

Feminist literature can be invigorating and illuminating, broadening the perspective and shedding light on the common denominators of the female experience.

And feminist organizations, such as the National Organization of Women (which has local chapters in most cities) and the National Women's Health Network (to name but two) can be valuable resource and support agencies, as well as avenues of action and participation.

One of the most positive aspects of feminist thinking is the pride it engenders in being a female, in valuing those unequaled qualities which are so unique to the female experience. Michael Polanyi (1958, p. 53) has said that "it is pathetic to watch the endless efforts — equipped with microscopy and chemistry, with mathematics and electronics — to reproduce a single violin of the kind the half-literate Stradivarius turned out as a matter of routine more than 200 years ago." Of course, the nurse is not a half-literate creature. However, in the "art" of her nursing role, she can proudly turn to those "feminine" qualities which have for so long and with such inaccuracy been demeaned — the "traditional" one-to-one relating with people, her capacity for empathy, the giving, compassionate, nurturing side of her nature. What better way to counteract, to humanize "modern" medicine, with its CAT scans and radio-immune assays, its computerized chemistry analyses and mechanized staffs?

If political action is a power of one kind, then valuing oneself as a woman is power of another kind. Feminism teaches this. Nursing must begin to consider the "feminine" aspect of our profession in a positive way. The nurturing, caretaking, empathic facets of our nature must be the basis on which we predicate our theories, our actions, and our very *raison d'etre*.

ADVERTISING & MARKETING — PROBLEM #4

I remember hearing a story about "the greatest advertising coup in history." Apparently, an advertising firm was hired to formulate a way to sell Alka Seltzer. A clever jingle writer composed a tune to which the words "Plop, plop, fizz, fizz, oh what a relief it is" were sung. Anticipated sales doubled — and, to this day, continue to be twice what they might have been — because people believed that, in order to get the "relief" they sought, they had to take two Alka Seltzers ("plop, plop") instead of the one tablet that would do the trick. How amazing: The ability to sell people something — even something they don't need — just with an inventive and catchy sales approach!

Of course, our entire economy is fueled by advertising and marketing. Billions are spent on cosmetics, largely the function of the "creative" Madison Avenue ability to convince women that they need this or that product in order to be attractive, desirable, sexy or just plain acceptable. Mail-order catalogues generate huge incomes selling people items (and many times gimmicks) which they could live an entire lifetime without. Of course, advertising also serves to illuminate people about the things they do need. The sales of everything from cars to appliances to homes to leisure gear to reading material *ad infinitum* — all depend upon advertising and marketing.

In today's world, even universities advertise their virtues and hospitals try to lure both nurses and doctors with advertisements featuring attractive salary and benefit offers.

Now that the rest of the professional world has caught on to the power of advertising and marketing, a proliferation of ads featuring accounting firms, chiropractic and dentistry practices, and law services fills the air waves and and television screen and occupies a good deal of space in the print media.

However, the advertising and marketing of nurses is nowhere to be found. To be sure, nurses have independent practices, in midwifery, in psychotherapy, as clinical nurse specialists in a variety of areas. They have skills in management, in community liaison work, in teaching. They conduct CPR classes and join life-saving units. But, in spite of their education, their clinical experience, their independent status, and their proven skills and talents in a variety of areas, the public's "image" of a nurse remains fixated in the past or wedded to the current images which movies and television have portrayed. In these depictions, the nurse is either toting a bed pan or shaking down a thermometer or she is the wicked Nurse Ratchet of moviedom or the machinating plotter on the soap opera or, as a final insult, she is the seductive, hare brained floozy portrayed on greeting cards.

Where is the nurse who imparts information, who reacts coolly and effectively in an emergency, who teaches pre-operative patients,who delivers a baby, who diagnoses and treats a depressed patient, who lobbies a state senator, who runs a critical care unit, who performs bedside nursing of the highest order, who assists in complicated surgery or diagnostic procedures, who saves a life?

We know she is there. We *are* these nurses. What to do?

ADVERTISING & MARKETING — SOLUTION #4

Nurses must put their own best foot forward. I remember a conversation I had just after becoming a certified childbirth instructor in 1979. When the subject of how to attract clients arose, it was clear that the consensus of the people I was speaking with thought that advertising was "unprofessional." Since their arguments were not convincing, I decided to embark on what Norman Mailer would call "Advertisements for Myself." Although I had left the delivery room where I had been employed for almost three years, I wrote a letter, not only to the doctors I had worked with, but also to a long list of doctors I had never met, from the Yellow Pages of my phone book. In the letter, I cited my delivery room experience, my accreditation in a nationally recognized childbirth association, a brief synopsis of the course I would be teaching, the geographical convenience of my home (where I teach) to the hospitals they worked in and to most of their own clientele, the advantages of small classes to this particular clientele, and some personal attributes that I thought would appeal to them. The return I got was about 4-5 percent, less than I had anticipated, but creditable according to the business people I talked to. However, that small percentage "put me on the map," so to speak, and allowed the "word-of-mouth" which is so vital to any business enterprise to happen more quickly than if I had not advertised. In addition, I hung advertisements in local supermarkets and spoke at local forums. In no time, it seemed, my practice began to flourish — and, as a bonus, I became a resource person (sometimes voluntary, sometimes in a paid capacity) to nurses and other women and men who wanted to establish independent enterprises.

Then, as now, I could not see how the advertising and marketing I did for myself is or was in any way unprofessional. In fact, it seems that everyone involved has benefitted — my clients, the doctors, the other people I advised, and me.

I have known other nurses who, catching the entrepreneurial spirit, have parlayed their background in nursing into profitable ventures. One runs a CPR company, teaching large corporations the techniques of cardio-pulmonary resuscitation. Another runs workshops in various industries in which she teaches techniques for better communication and for stress reduction. Another has started a business doing check-ups and health teaching for insurance companies. Another has started a private day-care center. And yet another has started a holistic healthcare practice. All of these nurses advertised and marketed themselves, using their nursing backgrounds to establish their credentials, their credibility and their authority.

But, unfortunately, the actions of a few do not speak for the many. We must have a national advertising campaign, perhaps sponsored by the American Nurses Association, which tells the American public who we are, what we do and how vital is our contribution to the American healthcare system. We must be portrayed in all of our variety, our breadth and our depth. And, we must be proud to advertise and market ourselves, to let the public at large know that we feel dignity in the choice of career we have made, that we are educated, that we are skilled, that we are multi-faceted in our talents, that we know our own worth and that we won't be undersold!

BUSINESS & LAW — PROBLEM #5

When nurses go into the hospital environment, they find themselves in the middle of a business armed with few, if any, business skills. Just as in the case of people who enter industry, they are called upon to punch a time clock, adhere to "company" regulations, deal with "higher-ups," and execute their jobs. Frequently, they find themselves in the middle of questionable practices (i.e., being asked to work "a little" overtime with no pay; to compensate for absent co-workers, even if the understaffing clearly endangers patients; adhering to sexist clothing codes, etc.) that demand at least a rudimentary familiarity with the law. Unknowledgeable and often intimidated, the nurse is placed in a compromised position, unable to challenge existing policies or defend her rights.

BUSINESS & LAW — SOLUTION #5

Nursing schools should encourage nurses (for credit) to do field work in the business and law setting. Even half a semester of such experience would familiarize the nurse with the internal workings of those respective settings, equip her with the tools to deal with the kinds of problems she will be confronted with when she enters the hospital.

In the hospital, nurses must insist that they be invited to seminars and meetings which focus upon these subjects. In addition, nurses must take advantage of the many seminars given around the country that directly address the business and/or legal issues which they encounter. Many of these seminars are given by nurses for nurses — many are given by people from the business and law community.

The purpose of gathering this type of information is empowerment. Knowledge not only diminishes the anxiety which arises when people find themselves in unfamiliar or threatening situations, it also endows people with a sense of their own authority, a sense that they are not victims — but, rather, that they are full, aware participants in the events of their lives.

PSYCHOLOGY — PROBLEM #6

The Talmud says, "We do not see things the way they are. We see things the way we are." Because our view of the world is limited to our own perspective and our own experience, it is easy to see how a person who has been devalued comes to devalue herself. She will see things through the jaded prism of her own vision — and not "as they are." In the same way, a person whose life experience has been fraught with anger and disappointment will see the world not as a benevolent and caring place, but as one which holds potential threats. Even in the absence of evidence, that person will see things not as they are, but as she is. Ultimately, the best chance we all have to change the things in our lives that displease us is to change ourselves.

I once attended a seminar in which the moderator explained that there are only three ways that people truly change: through a brush with death, through a profoundly religious experience or through psychotherapy. I cannot attest to the validity of this theory, but I do believe that people who want to change, can.

Of course, it would be ideal if children were not raised in sexist environments or in settings which devalue females. It would also be wonderful if females and males could be perceived according to who they are, and not according to the still rigid "gender roles" that determine so much of modern life. However, before these global changes come to pass, the best we can do is to be aware of our own implication in the lives we lead — and to strive for the kinds of personal and societal changes which would bring them about.

PSYCHOLOGY — SOLUTION #6

For those contemplating psychotherapy, there are several schools which might be considered:

Psychotherapy: Sometimes called psychodynamic psychotherapy, this method attributes emotional problems to unconscious internal conflicts. Usually a lengthy process in which childhood traumas are explored, dreams analyzed, and transference phenomena given important interpretive meaning, psychotherapy explores symptoms by identifying the pattern of defense and the developmental history of the symptoms. In this type of psychotherapy, change is usually slower in coming than in some other types of therapy. It is for the patient who is highly motivated to change and who is interested in learning of the symbolic nature of her or his symptoms.

Cognitive Therapy: This treatment focuses on altering troublesome thoughts. Developed by Aaron Beck, a psychiatrist at the University of Pennsylvania, it is predicated on the theory that the ways in which we think about ourselves and the world affect how we feel and behave. When the therapist points out to the patient his or her cognitive errors and then teaches methods in rethinking, both feelings and behavior are altered.

Behavioral Therapy: Based on Pavlovian conditioning, this therapy operates on the premise that behavior is affected by either positive or negative reinforcement. The goal is to get patients to learn new and more appropriate responses. This type of therapy is particularly effective in treating phobias and other behavioral problems which interfere with normal daily living.

Interpersonal Therapy: This therapy attributes psychological problems to faulty relationships. Frequently, it
includes family members who, through the therapeutic milieu, learn in which ways their behavior influences the existing problem.

These are but a few of the myriad of types of therapies which exist. In addition, there are group therapies,
support groups, psychodrama (in which emotional situations are acted out), consciousness-raising groups and cri-
sis-intervention therapy — again, to name but a few.

And so, when it comes to "Solutions," there is surely
an abundance of possibilities — ranging from the personal
to the political, from the academic to the public sector —
for the nurse who feels that she "can't take it anymore"
and that she is tired of the Nurse Abuse which pervades
her life.

The current crisis in nursing — indeed, the future
of nursing — can be resolved if we invoke the philosophy
of "Nurse-Heal Thyself." It is time to turn our full attention, not to the image we have had, but to the substance
that we have. Nursing must take a hard and critical look
at itself, acknowledge its flaws, and then embark on revolutionary measures of change.

Happily, many of these changes have already begun. It is up to us — the nurses of America — to see that
the momentum continues.

References

Brown, Sharon. (1985). "Perspective on why nurses should earn doctorates in nursing." *Perspectives in Psychiatric Care.* No. 1, Vol. XXIII.

Corea, Gena. (1977). *The hidden malpractice: How American medicine treats women as patients and professionals.* New York: William Morrow & Co.

Ehrenreich, Barbara., & English, Deirdre. (1973). *Witches, midwives and nurses.* New York: The Feminist Press.

Gilligan, Carol. (1982). *In a different voice: Psychological theory and women's development.* Cambridge: Harvard University Press.

Hewlett, Sylvia Ann. (1986). *A lesser life: The myth of women's liberation in America.* New York: Warner Books.

Kuhn, Thomas S. (1970). *The structure of scientific revolutions.* Chicago: University of Chicago Press.

Polanyi, Michael. (1958). *Personal knowledge.* Chicago: University of Chicago Press.

Riehl, Joan P., & Callista, Roy. (1980). *Conceptual model for nursing practice.* Norwalk, Connecticut: Appleton-Century-Crofts.

Swirsky, Joan. (1988). "Nurse-heal thyself", *The New York Times.* May 22.

U.S. News and World Report.   Dentzer, Susan. (1988). "Calling the shots in health care: The nursing shortage points up a growing turf war between doctors and nurses."

Chapter Ten

Nurse's
Bill of Rights

Nursing warrants fair and
equitable compensation
as is given to other
professions with
comparable education,
expertise
and responsibility.

It is nursing's privilege to consider and implement collective bargaining in order to secure and resolve the issue of comparable worth.

Nurses should receive
direct reimbursement in
the form of
fee-for-service for the
comprehensive and skilled
care they provide.

Nurses must have the right to refuse re-assignment to patient care areas foreign to their specialty of practice, for nurses must be regarded as unique practitioners. Nurses are not interchangeable.

Nurses must be respected and valued by colleagues as integral and vital members of the healthcare team, their assessments and recommendations considered essential in formulating the strategies of patient care.

Nurses employed in a bureaucratic institution are entitled to the respect and support from administration regarding issues concerning delivery of patient care.

Nurses must be able to actively participate in formulating policies that directly affect them and patient care.

Employers are obligated to establish an environment in which nurses are actively involved in determining the standards of practice necessary for implementing quality patient care.

Employers must provide
an adequate amount of
ancillary services to
abolish time spent with
non-nursing duties.

Nurses must be guaranteed a technologically efficient atmosphere in which to function, enabling them to maximize the time required to delivery direct patient care.

Financial support must
be available for the
enhancement of clinical
knowledge and attainment
of educational goals.

An effective mechanism
of disciplinary action
must be established
in which nurses,
as patient advocates,
may report professional
incompetence and
situations that compromise
patient care.

TO ORDER ADDITIONAL COPIES
OF
NURSE ABUSE
IMPACT AND RESOLUTION

Editors

Laura Gasparis RN, MA, CEN, CCRN
Joan Swirsky RN, MS, CS

with
Ten Contributing Authors

Book Price $19.95 plus $3.00 shipping & handling

Mail the form below along with a check or money order for $22.95 to:
Power Publications
56 McArthur Avenue
Staten Island, New York 10312
or call
1-800-331-6534 and charge to MC or Visa

Power Publications
56 McArthur Avenue Staten Island, New York 10312

Name _____ Specialty _____

Address _____

City _____ State _____ Zip _____

☐ Check/MO

☐ Visa # _____

☐ MasterCard # _____

☐ Signature _____

Payment must accompany this order form.

THE NIGHTINGALE CONSPIRACY:

NURSING COMES TO POWER
IN THE 21st CENTURY

by Karilee Halo Shames RN, Ph.D

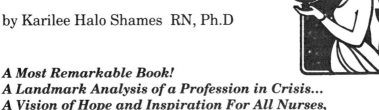

A Most Remarkable Book!
A Landmark Analysis of a Profession in Crisis...
A Vision of Hope and Inspiration For All Nurses,
All Women and All Health Care Consumers.

Finally, the book every nurse has been waiting for — the story of nursing in its past, present, and FUTURE! Have you ever wondered where we nurses came from originally? What happened to us over the centuries to explain our present plight?

Have you ever stopped to examine the differences between the education we've received and the jobs we're doing in hospitals? Are you confused?

This author, Karilee Halo Shames, was too. She couldn't understand the inner conflict she experienced in her nursing endeavors, or the outer conflict, until she was asked to leave a position and stumbled upon some shocking realizations — and she has dedicated her professional life to awakening us all to the **power we possess to change the system.**

Topics discussed in this unusual book range from our history (herstory!) to codependency, from self-esteem issues to professional recognition, from societal expectations to unity and support. It discusses the very issues which we ourselves have often ignored, at a great expense.

THE TIME HAS COME TO GO BEYOND PROBLEMS,
INTO *SOLUTIONS.*

The author now tours the U.S., speaking her truth as a nursing therapist and advocate. She has examined the past and envisions a healthier future, and now invites YOU to participate in the healthiest movement around...

THE NIGHTINGALE CONSPIRACY

The Nightingale Conspiracy

Book Price $19.95 plus $3.00 shipping & handling

Mail the form below along with a check or money order for $22.95 to:

Power Publications
56 McArthur Avenue
Staten Island, New York 10312
or call
1-800-331-6534 and charge to MC or Visa

Power Publications
56 McArthur Avenue Staten Island, New York 10312

Name _____ Specialty _____

Address _____

City _____ State _____ Zip _____

☐ Check/MO

☐ Visa # _____

☐ MasterCard # _____

☐ Signature _____

Payment must accompany this order form.

---

*The author, Karilee Halo Shames, is a clinical specialist in psychiatric nursing with advanced studies in holistic health. She writes her own column in two nursing magazines, has published many nursing and non-nursing articles, was co-founder of a national nurses support network in 1977 and presently is director of her own speaking and consulting firm, **Nurse Empowerment Workshops & Services.** She is eager to serve the needs of nurses through her writing and speaking endeavors.*

It is clear that the time has come for a **Revolution!**

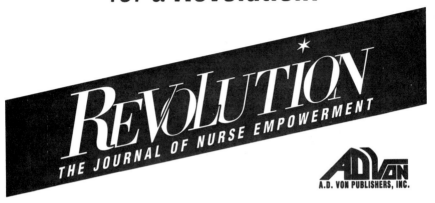

A.D. VON PUBLISHERS, INC.

Let us move forward with a creative mind and a heightened consciousness—for we have been submerged too long in a situation in which these qualities have been unrecognized.

Let us act upon and transform our profession of nursing.

Let us break the historically vicious cycle of powerlessness. Knowledge and influence are power. Nurses need more power! We need the opportunity to speak about ourselves in ways that heighten our pride, nurture our self-esteem and convey the uniqueness of our chosen path.

Let us not be victims! Rather, let us increase our awareness as to those social and historical forces that have traditionally cast us in a subservient role. Let us examine the effects that our nursing education and our society have had on the nurse in her everyday work environment. Let us discern those social, political and philosophical influences that have resulted in the victimization of nurses, and let us explore the consequences of being female in a patriarchal society.

Let us stop agonizing and begin organizing. Let us generate in the reader a commitment to the development of professional power, outlining strategies and giving nurses more ammunition to achieve power in both their personal and professional lives and in their work environment.

Problems demand solutions. The solutions to nursing problems lie in self-awareness, personal activism and...In **Revolution – The Journal of Nurse Empowerment!**